# Intraoperative MRI in Functional Neurosurgery

*Guest Editors*

DANIEL A. LIM, MD, PhD
PAUL S. LARSON, MD

# NEUROSURGERY CLINICS OF NORTH AMERICA

www.neurosurgery.theclinics.com

*Consulting Editors*
ANDREW T. PARSA, MD, PhD
PAUL C. McCORMICK, MD, MPH

April 2009 • Volume 20 • Number 2

SAUNDERS an imprint of ELSEVIER, Inc.

**W.B. SAUNDERS COMPANY**
*A Division of Elsevier Inc.*

1600 John F. Kennedy Blvd. • Suite 1800 • Philadelphia, PA 19103-2899

http://www.theclinics.com

**NEUROSURGERY CLINICS OF NORTH AMERICA Volume 20, Number 2**
**April 2009 ISSN 1042-3680, ISBN-13: 978-1-4377-1573-6, ISBN-10: 1-4377-1573-7**

Editor: Ruth Malwitz
Developmental Editor: Donald Mumford

*Neurosurgery Clinics of North America* (ISSN 1042-3680) is published quarterly by Elsevier Inc., 360 Park Avenue South, New York, NY 10010-1710. Months of issue are January, April, July, and October. Business and Editorial Offices: 1600 John F. Kennedy Blvd., Suite 1800, Philadelphia, PA 19103-2899. Customer Service Office: 11830 Westline Industrial Drive, St. Louis, MO 63146. Periodicals postage paid at New York, NY, and additional mailing offices. Subscription prices are $274.00 per year (US individuals), $438.00 per year (US institutions), $300.00 per year (Canadian individuals), $535.00 per year (Canadian institutions), $383.00 per year (international individuals), $535.00 per year (international institutions), $138.00 per year (US students), and $189.00 per year (international students). International air speed delivery is included in all *Clinics* subscription prices. All prices are subject to change without notice. **POSTMASTER:** Send address changes to *Neurosurgery Clinics of North America*, Elsevier Periodicals Customer Service, 11830 Westline Industrial Drive, St. Louis, MO 63146. **Customer Service: 1-800-654-2452 (US and Canada). From outside the US and Canada, call: 1-314-453-7041. Fax: 1-314-453-5170. E-mail: JournalsCustomerService-usa@elsevier.com (for print support) and journalsonlinesupport-usa@elsevier.com (for online support).**

*Reprints.* For copies of 100 or more, of articles in this publication, please contact the Commercial Reprints Department, Elsevier Inc., 360 Park Avenue South, New York, NY 10010-1710. Tel. (212) 633-3812; Fax: (212) 462-1935; E-mail: reprints@elsevier.com.

*Neurosurgery Clinics of North America* is covered in *MEDLINE/PubMed (Index Medicus)*, *EMBASE/Excerpta Medica, and Current Contents/Clinical Medicine (CC/CM)*.

Printed and bound by CPI Group (UK) Ltd, Croydon, CR0 4YY

# Contributors

## GUEST EDITORS

**DANIEL A. LIM, MD, PhD**
Assistant Professor, Director of Restorative
Neurosurgery, Member, Eli and Edythe Broad
Center of Regeneration Medicine and Stem
Cell Research at UCSF, Department of
Neurological Surgery, University of California,
San Francisco; Staff Neurosurgeon,
Neurosurgical Section, Surgical Service,
San Francisco Veterans Affairs Medical
Center, Department of Veterans Affairs,
San Francisco, California

**PAUL S. LARSON, MD**
Associate Clinical Professor, Department of
Neurological Surgery, University of California
San Francisco, San Francisco; Chief,
Neurosurgical Section, Surgical Service,
San Francisco Veteran Affairs Medical Center,
Department of Veteran Affairs, San Francisco,
California

## AUTHORS

**K.S. BANKIEWICZ, MD, PhD**
Kinetics Foundation Chair in Translational
Research and Professor, Department
of Neurological Surgery, Laboratory for
Molecular Therapeutics, University of
California San Francisco, San Francisco,
California

**CAROL J. BARBRE, BS**
Vice President Product Management,
SurgiVision, Inc., Irvine, California

**SERGIO D. BERGESE, MD**
Assistant Clinical Professor, Director
of Neuroanesthesia, Department of
Anesthesiology and Neurological Surgery,
The Ohio State University Medical Center,
Columbus, Ohio

**PETER M. BLACK, MD, PhD**
Franc D Ingraham Professor, Department
of Neurosurgery, Harvard Medical School,
Brigham and Women's Hospital, Boston,
Massachusetts

**LUTZ DÖRNER, MD**
Department of Neurosurgery, University
Hospital Schleswig-Holstein, Campus Kiel,
Kiel, Germany

**J.R. FORSAYETH, PhD**
Department of Neurological Surgery,
Laboratory for Molecular Therapeutics,
University of California San Francisco,
San Francisco, California

**ALEXANDRA J. GOLBY, MD**
Assistant Professor, Department
of Neurosurgery, Harvard Medical School,
Brigham and Women's Hospital, Boston,
Massachusetts

**WALTER A. HALL, MD, MBA**
Professor, Department of Radiology, Hennepin
County Medical Center, Minneapolis,
Minnesota; and Department of Neurosurgery,
State University of New York, Upstate Medical
University, Syracuse, New York

**THOMAS JOHNSTON, MD**
Department of Neurological Surgery,
Resident, University of Louisville,
Louisville, Kentucky

**PETER D. KIM, MD, PhD**
Resident, Department of Neurosurgery,
State University of New York,
Upstate Medical University, Syracuse,
New York

# Contributors

**PAUL S. LARSON, MD**
Associate Clinical Professor, Department of Neurological Surgery, University of California San Francisco, San Francisco; Chief, Neurosurgical Section, Surgical Service, San Francisco Veteran Affairs Medical Center, Department of Veteran Affairs, San Francisco, California

**DANIEL A. LIM, MD, PhD**
Assistant Professor, Director of Restorative Neurosurgery, Member, Eli and Edythe Broad Center of Regeneration Medicine and Stem Cell Research at UCSF, Department of Neurological Surgery, University of California, San Francisco; Staff Neurosurgeon, Neurosurgical Section, Surgical Service, San Francisco Veterans Affairs Medical Center, Department of Veterans Affairs, San Francisco, California

**SHELLY LWU, MD, MSc**
Neurosurgery resident, Department of Clinical Neurosciences, University of Calgary, Calgary, Canada

**ALASTAIR J. MARTIN, PhD**
Associate Professor, Department of Radiology and Biomedical Imaging, University of California San Francisco, San Francisco, California

**H. MAXIMILIAN MEHDORN, MD, PhD**
Department of Neurosurgery, University Hospital Schleswig-Holstein, Campus Kiel, Kiel, Germany

**JOHN M.K. MISLOW, MD, PhD**
Department of Neurosurgery, Harvard Medical School, Brigham and Women's Hospital, Children's Hospital Boston, Boston, Massachusetts

**KAREN MOELLER, MD**
Department of Neurological Surgery, University of Louisville, Louisville, Kentucky; Department of Pediatric Radiology, Kosair Childrens' Hospital, Division of Pediatric Neuroradiology, Louisville, Kentucky; Norton Healthcare, Louisville, Kentucky

**THOMAS M. MORIARTY, MD**
Department of Neurological Surgery, University of Louisville, Louisville, Kentucky; Norton Healthcare, Louisville, Kentucky; Department of Neurological Surgery, Associate Professor of Neurological Surgery, Chief–Pediatric Neurosurgery, Kosair Childrens' Hospital, Louisville, Kentucky

**ROBERT MOSER**
Norton Healthcare, Louisville, Kentucky

**ARYA NABAVI, MD**
Department of Neurosurgery, University Hospital Schleswig-Holstein, Campus Kiel, Kiel, Germany

**ERIKA G. PUENTE, MD**
Post Doctoral Researcher, Department of Anesthesiology, The Ohio State University Medical Center, Columbus, Ohio

**R.M. RICHARDSON, MD, PhD**
Resident, Department of Neurological Surgery, Laboratory for Molecular Therapeutics, University of California San Francisco, San Francisco, California

**JOSHUA ROSKOM, BA**
Department of Neurological Surgery, University of California San Fransisco, San Francisco, California

**ANDREAS M. STARK, MD**
Department of Neurosurgery, University Hospital Schleswig-Holstein, Campus Kiel, Kiel, Germany

**PHILIP A. STARR, MD, PhD**
Associate Professor, Department of Neurological Surgery, University of California San Francisco, San Francisco, California

**GARNETTE R. SUTHERLAND, MD**
Professor of Neurosurgery, Department of Clinical Neurosciences, University of Calgary, Calgary; Director of Seaman Family MR Research Centre, University of Calgary, Calgary, Alberta, Canada

**ANDRZEJ SWISTOWSKI, PhD**
Postdoctoral Researcher, Buck Institute
for Age Research, Novato,
California

**CHARLES L. TRUWIT, MD**
Professor, Department of Radiology,
University of Minnesota Medical School;
and Department of Radiology,
Hennepin County Medical Center,
Minneapolis, Minnesota

**V. VARENIKA, BS**
Laboratory for Molecular Therapeutics,
Department of Neurological Surgery, University
of California San Francisco, San Francisco,
California

**XIANMIN ZENG, PhD**
Associate Professor, Director of the North Bay
California Institute for Regenerative Medicine
(CIRM) Shared Research Laboratory for Stem
Cells & Aging; Buck Institute for Age Research,
Novato, California

Contributors

ANDRZEJ SWISTOWSKI, PhD
Postdoctoral Researcher, Buck Institute
for Age Research, Novato,
California

CHARLES L. TRUWIT, MD
Professor, Department of Radiology,
University of Minnesota Medical School,
and Department of Radiology,
Hennepin County Medical Center,
Minneapolis, Minnesota

V. VALENKA, BS
Laboratory for Molecular Therapeutics,
Department of Neurological Surgery, University
of California San Francisco, San Francisco,
California

XIANMIN ZENG, PhD
Associate Professor, Director of the North Bay
California Institute for Regenerative Medicine
(CIRM) Shared Research Laboratory for Stem
Cells & Aging, Buck Institute for Age Research,
Novato, California

# Contents

in the integration of robotic technology into medicine. This article describes the development and clinical application of neuroArm, a magnetic resonance—compatible robot capable of both stereotaxy and microsurgery.

# Neurosurgery Clinics of North America

## THE CLINICS ARE NOW AVAILABLE ONLINE!

Access your subscription at:
**www.theclinics.com**

# Preface

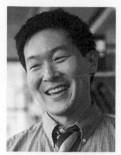 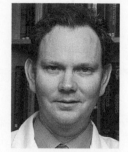

Daniel A. Lim, MD, PhD      Paul S. Larson, MD
*Guest Editors*

Imaging technologies have led to tremendous advancements in the field of neurosurgery, and this merging of imaging with surgical techniques is particularly evident in the recent developments of interventional or intraoperative magnetic resonance imaging (iMRI). Over the past 20 years, iMRI has evolved from a technique intended to improve the surgical outcome for brain tumor resections to one that is particularly well suited for the treatment of disorders in functional neurosurgery. As Guest Editors of this issue of *Neurosurgery Clinics of North America*, we have assembled a series of articles related to iMRI with topics spanning from the historical perspective of iMRI developments for brain tumor surgery, to the considerations of operating room safety and anesthesia, to technologic developments on both the hardware and software ends, to current uses for the treatment of Parkinson's disease, and concluding with two articles that look to the future of neurosurgery with iMRI for gene therapy and cell transplantation.

We designed this issue of *The Clinics* to be somewhat of a departure from the style of past issues. We intend this issue to broadly interest those in the fields of neurosurgery, neurology, and radiology, as these are the disciplines that will need to work together for the successful application of iMRI. We designed this issue to be highly visual, with the inclusion of many color figures. We thus hope that this relatively thin issue is visually appealing and intellectually approachable to scientists, physicians, and lay people alike.

One hope is that this issue will provide just enough technical detail to provide others with a basic "starting point" from which to begin designing a program of iMRI for functional neurosurgery. Another hope is that basic scientists who read this issue will gain a better understanding of the translational research issues, and in this way perhaps guide their own research. A final hope is that this issue of *The Clinics* will inspire others to dream of novel uses for the general approaches described herein.

Daniel A. Lim, MD, PhD
Paul S. Larson, MD

Neurosurgical Section, Surgical Service
San Francisco Veterans Affairs Medical Center
Department of Veterans Affairs
4150 Clement Street
San Francisco, CA 94121, USA

Department of Neurological Surgery
University of California San Francisco
505 Parnassus Avenue, Room M779
San Francisco, CA 94143, USA

E-mail addresses:
LimD@neurosurg.ucsf.edu (D.A. Lim)
LarsonP@neurosurg.ucsf.edu (P.S. Larson)

doi:10.1016/j.nec.2009.04.014
1042-3680/09/$ – see front matter

# Origins of Intraoperative MRI

John M.K. Mislow, MD, PhD, Alexandra J. Golby, MD*,
Peter M. Black, MD, PhD

**KEYWORDS**

- Intraoperative • MRI • Functional • Neurosurgery
- Brain • Tumor • Epilepsy

Successful neurosurgical procedures hinge on the accurate targeting of regions of interest. Resection of brain tumors is enhanced by the surgeon's ability to accurately define margins. Epileptic foci are identified by coregistration of functional and antatomic information, and stereotactic targets must be pinpointed with submillimetric accuracy for surgical efficacy. Specialized neuronavigational tools have been developed over the last 20 years to assist surgeons in these endeavors; the development of MRI-guided navigation systems represents a significant improvement in the surgical treatment of various intracranial lesions. The ability for most intraoperative image guidance systems to remain faithful to the anatomy once the cranium has been opened remains problematic, however. "Brain shift," the term applied to the dynamic change that intracranial anatomy undergoes after craniotomy, burr hole placement, drainage of cerebrospinal fluid, or resection of a lesion, compromises the localization of neural structures in space relative to where they were when preoperative images were acquired (**Fig. 1**).[1–8] Gliomas also pose a particular challenge to surgeons because many of these tumors (particularly low-grade gliomas) do not possess distinct capsules. As a result, even well-trained human eyes are incapable of discerning where the border of the lesion ends and viable brain begins. This uncertainty leads to two problems: (1) inadequate resection secondary to the surgeon stopping at what appears to be grossly abnormal tissue (so as to avoid neurologic damage) and (2) neurologic damage caused by aggressive surgery in which resection ends only when clearly normal brain tissue is visualized.

Only intraoperatively acquired images can provide neurosurgeons with the information needed to perform real-time, image-guided surgery. Uncertainty is reduced significantly when the surgeon places an instrument at the edge of what is believed to be the resection cavity, and a small nodule of tumor is immediately identified by intraoperative imaging. Avoidance and preservation of eloquent cortex such as motor, speech, and visual areas depend on precise identification of these regions during the procedure. The boundary between tumor and viable neural tissue is often difficult to see with the naked eye, so the superimposition of functional MRI, diffusion tensor imaging, and awake cortical mapping images eliminates a surgeon's uncertainty in determining tumor boundary and shifting brain structures. This leads to surgeons achieving maximal lesion resection while minimizing untoward neurologic sequelae. Maximal lesion resection is a principal goal in tumor resection because abundant evidence indicates that a more complete resection directly impacts the survival time of patients with low- and high-grade gliomas.[9–18]

## ORIGINS OF INTRAOPERATIVE MRI: 0.5T OPEN-CONFIGURATION PROTOTYPE

The origin of iMRI for neurosurgery was the Magnetic Resonance Therapy (MRT) Unit at

This article was supported by the following grants: NIH F32-NS061483-01A1 (JM). NIH P01-CA67165, U41-RR 019,703, K08 NS48063-01, and the Brain Science Foundation (AG).
Department of Neurosurgery, Harvard Medical School, Brigham and Women's Hospital, 75 Francis Street, Boston, MA 02115, USA
* Corresponding author.
*E-mail address:* agolby@partners.org (A.J. Golby).

Neurosurg Clin N Am 20 (2009) 137–146
doi:10.1016/j.nec.2009.04.002
1042-3680/09/$ – see front matter © 2009 Published by Elsevier Inc.

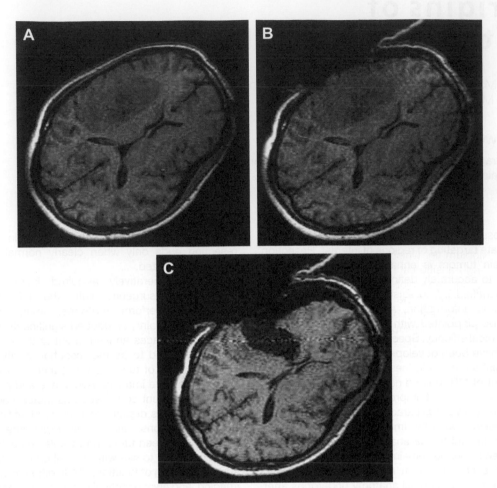

**Fig. 1.** Brain shift. (*A*) T1-weighted axial MRI before craniotomy. (*B*) Same axial plane MRI after craniotomy performed. (*C*) MRI after lesion resection. Note the significant shift of intracranial contents after craniotomy, cerebrospinal fluid drainage, and lesion resection.

Brigham and Women's Hospital (BWH) in Boston, Massachusetts. It began as a collaborative project among four groups: Ferenc Jolesz of the Department of Radiology at BWH, engineers at General Electric Medical Systems (Milwaukee, Wisconsin), the neurosurgical service at BWH with Dr. Peter Black as head, and the department of otorhinolaryngology with Marvin Fried as director. Throughout the late 1980s, these physicians and scientists collaborated in the development of an open-configuration MRI scanner that allowed surgery to be performed with concurrent intraoperative image guidance. At the time of inception, the closed-configuration of conventional MRI systems precluded direct access to the patient; therefore, fundamental changes in magnet and coil design and display methods were necessary to fully realize the concept of iMRI. This concept was a radical departure from MR physics of the time, with the magnetic field highest in the space between the double donut.

Early interventional procedures in an open MRI system were performed in a low-field imager by Gronemeyer and colleagues.[19,20] This system provided access to patients through a horizontal gap in its magnet. Access was significantly limited, however, and open surgeries that required full access to patients were impractical. Based on this information, after discussing several alternative designs, a "double donut" magnet system that would allow free access to patients within the magnetic field was chosen by BWH for development.[21] The initial research and development phase came to fruition in 1994 with the completion and installation of a prototype midfield intraoperative MRI system (GE 0.5-T Signa SP) unit at the BWH (**Fig. 2**).[22–24]

Direct access to patients was achieved by the construction of two vertically oriented superconducting magnets with coils in separate but communicating cryocoolers. This design results in a vertical gap between the coils through which

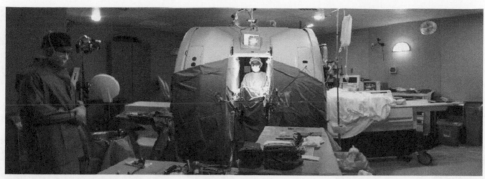

**Fig. 2.** The MRT unit at BWH. The General Electric Signa 0.5T iMRI is an open-configuration "double donut" system that allows the surgeon to operate between each superconductive magnet coil (pictured).

patients can be fully accessed during image acquisition. Niobium tin, which has a maximum superconducting transition at higher temperatures than the more common niobium titanium, allows for sufficient cooling of the coils and thermal shield with cryocooler assembly, which eliminates the need for liquid helium coolant. This design resulted in a significantly increased area of patient access: the modified magnet provides a spherical imaging volume 30 cm in diameter and a 56-cm wide area of patient access, allowing surgeons and first assistants to be positioned on either side of patients.[21] In addition to the wide patient access area, the configuration of the "double-donut" magnet allows the position of patients within the imager to be flexible; the table can be inserted into the magnet along two orthogonal axes ("end docked" and "side docked"), which allows convenient access to different areas of anatomy. Because of the open configuration of the MRT, surgeons can perform various percutaneous, interventional, endoscopic, or open surgical procedures while standing or sitting and simultaneously viewing intraoperatively obtained MRI displayed on monitors placed in the gap of the magnet.

Many challenges needed to be met during the original implementation of iMRI, including the development of MRI-compatible equipment, instruments, and various tools along with the integration of the intraoperative display of images, the audiovisual communication among the team members, and the interactive manipulation of image data.

The initial phase of the iMRI project was slowed down by the unavailability of MR-compatible surgical instruments. In many cases, extensive changes were required to adapt instruments and equipment to the unique electromagnetic environment.[25–28] Many ferromagnetic surgical instruments were replaced by titanium, providing the essential capabilities required for craniotomies without becoming a ballistic hazard. Several metallic instruments that were not ferromagnetic still caused a substantial artifact when placed near a target within the imaging field of view and could not be used. An early problem was the headholder, which had to be firm, nonferromagnetic, and flexible. It was possible to create a headholder similar to the Mayfield device made of high performance plastic, but it took many months. The next challenge was the power drill; for more than a year, the only procedures that could be done were biopsies because there was no way to turn a craniotomy flap. The Midas Rex Corporation (Medtronic, Minniapolis, Minnesota) finally was able to create a nonferromagnetic drill. The operating microscope was the third major device to be created; it was possible to create a plastic microscope with nonferromagnetic joints that, although simple, was adequate. Finally, we were able to develop a bipolar coagulator whose current would not interfere with the magnetic field. Each of these technologic developments took 6 to 12 months to complete, but gradually it was possible to do surgery in the intraoperative GE Signa system just as readily as in a routine operating room. Anesthesia and patient monitoring systems that did not emit any electronic noise and could function during a scan were developed and installed within the MRT suite[29]; fortunately, they had been created for performing pediatric MR imaging under anesthesia.

The development of imaging during surgery led to the "Surgical Planning Laboratory" at BWH. The occurrence of surgically induced volumetric deformations known as brain shift has been well established. There were no detailed analyses, however, of the changes that occur during surgery. As a result, Gering and colleagues[30] at BWH developed a volumetric display software (3D Slicer; www.slicer.org) that allowed quantitative analysis of the degree and direction of brain shift (**Fig. 3**). For 25 patients, multiple intraoperative volumetric image acquisitions were

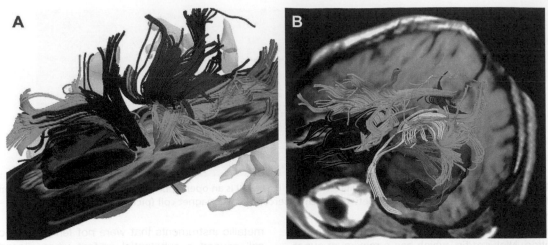

**Fig. 3.** Intraoperative colocalization using iMRI images and 3-D Slicer software. (*A*) Tumor, functional MRI, and diffusion tensor imaging are colocalized with standard MRI. (*B*) After craniotomy is performed, 3-D Slicer compensates for brain shift, allowing surgeons to visualize not only shift of gross neuroanatomy but also functional regions and white matter tracts.

extensively evaluated. It was found that brain shift is a continuous dynamic process that evolves differently in distinct brain regions. The authors concluded that only serial imaging or continuous data acquisition can provide consistently accurate image guidance.[30,31] Further refinements in tracking intraoperative brain deformation were performed in a pilot study by Archip and colleagues in 2008.[32]

The combination of the 0.5-T iMRI and three-dimensional slicer transformed the MRT into an exceptionally effective tool for neurosurgeons. Since the first craniotomy for brain tumor resection in 1996, more than 1000 craniotomies for intracranial tumor resection have taken place in the MRT (40% low-grade gliomas, 50% high-grade gliomas, and 10% other intracranial lesions such as metastases, meningiomas, and vascular malformations).[33,34] In most patients with brain tumor operated on in the MRT, resection rates of 80% or more were achieved.[10] This percentage reinforces the value of iMRI in extension of lifespan of patients, because patients with subtotal tumor resection are at a higher risk of recurrence and death compared with patients with gross total tumor removal.

## EXPANDING THE SCOPE OF OPEN-CONFIGURATION INTRAOPERATIVE MRI

The BWH MRT was the original iMRI system but it was by no means the last. Because of the specialized nature of the equipment, the entire MRT suite needed to be custom-made to accommodate the scanner. Room shielding, coolant,

and power consumption were only a few of the expensive and high-maintenance aspects of the MRT. iMRI had proven itself to be a powerful tool in the hands of neurosurgeons attempting to achieve maximal tumor resection while

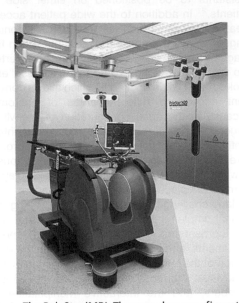

**Fig. 4.** The PoleStar iMRI. The open-bore configuration PoleStar N-20, despite its low-field 0.15T magnet, has allowed many institutions to take advantage of iMRI without completely remodeling their operative suite to accommodate a larger, high-field stationary iMRI. The Polestar is compact enough to be stored in a shielded room (pictured on the right side of the figure) when not in use. If a smaller room cannot be dedicated to storage, an in-suite "hangar" can be set up to shield the magnet when not in use. (*Courtesy of* Medtronic Navigation, Louisville, CO; with permission.)

preserving neurologic function, but how could institutions and practitioners take advantage of this technology without embarking on the expense of a major remodeling of their operative suite?

There were several answers, all driven by neurosurgeons. A major center was Erlangen, where Rudolph Fahlbusch helped to develop multiple concepts of Siemens for intraoperative imaging. This system moved from a side-opening low field to a system in which a table rotated into and out of a 1.5-T closed-bore magnet. Fahlbusch showed that for pituitary tumors and low-grade gliomas this system had a major advantage over other systems. A second answer was driven by the Israeli surgeon Moshe Hadani and his group.[35] Initially introduced in 2001 by Hadani and collagues,[35] the PoleStar (Medtronic Navigation, Louisville, Colorado) N-10 iMRI offered an open-configuration, portable 0.12-T magnet that required only modest remodeling of the operative suite. The device was stored in what amounted to a small

garage within the operating theater. The N-10's compact size and low magnetic footprint allowed units to be integrated into multiple institutions' conventional operating rooms. Despite a slightly increased time for induction of anesthesia and intubation, the units made a significant and positive impact on the safety and completeness of tumor resection in adult and pediatric intracranial procedures.[36–41] PoleStar recently introduced a higher-field (0.15 T) N-20 (**Fig. 4**), and initial evaluations confirm that the accuracy, versatility, and quality of this new-generation iMRI scanner are at least as good as the N-10. Clearly further clinical analysis of the accuracy on clinical cases using the N-20 is needed to confirm that these results will bear out in surgical reality.[36,37,42]

Other open-configuration iMRIs have since been developed. A 0.3-T horizontal iMRI by Hitachi at the University of Cincinnati[43,44] is a customized diagnostic iMRI, but the draping configuration does not lend itself to the sterile nature of neurosurgical interventions.

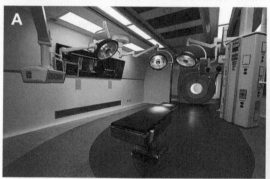
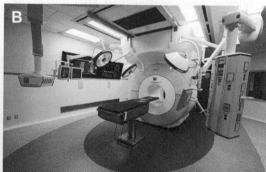
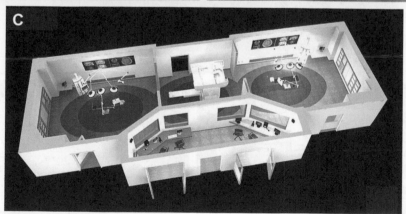

**Fig. 5.** The IMRIS iMRI. The IMRIS iMRI suite features a high-field, closed-bore magnet. (*A*) The IMRIS magnet in its storage room, shielding doors opened to show its relation to the operative suite when not in use. (*B*) The magnet has moved on its ceiling-mounted rails to its position over the region of the patient's head. The 1.5-T magnet can be brought from its park position in the storage room to a fully operational position within the operating room in less than 90 seconds, allowing for efficient scanning while still remaining unobtrusive. (*C*) An example of the IMRIS magnet serving two separate operating rooms. (The magnet can swivel 180° in the storage room to orient the working end toward the appropriate operating room.) (*Courtesy of* IMRIS, Inc., Winninpeg, Manitoba, Canada.)

## ORIGINS OF CLOSED-CONFIGURATION INTRAOPERATIVE MRI

A significant shortfall of the BWH MRT was the relatively low field offered by such a specialized system: the 0.5-T field did not yield image resolution comparable to contemporary diagnostic 1.5-T and 3-T MRI scanners. Initially, the basis of the double-donut design was that sacrifice of high-field imaging was acceptable if the patient did not have to be moved. This paradigm of imaging on demand proved to be efficient and effective over more than a decade. The field moved toward a paradigm of "in and out" imaging, however, primarily to enable the use of more off-the-shelf scanners. Surgical teams have developed protocols for moving patients in and out of the scanner that are relatively rapid and efficient. Methods to maintain patient registration data throughout the procedure were developed using an integrated overhead navigation camera or fixed markers on patients.[45,46] As a result of these findings, it was felt that the next iteration that should evolve from the original open-configuration MRT would be developed from a high-field, closed-bore system.

Consequently, several static closed-bore 1.5-T and 3-T systems have been installed in a growing number of institutions.[46,47] They are essentially hybrid systems that can be used for imaging or surgery.

The IMRIS system was developed by a neurosurgeon, Dr. Garnette Sutherland of Calgary, Alberta, Canada. This system offers a unique intraoperative rail-mounted system in which the scanner is brought to patients (**Fig. 5**). By enabling the MR system to move to patients, the system allows for improved surgical work-flow and enhanced patient safety in the surgical environment. The 70-cm bore 1.5-T magnet is able to move from room to room via a ceiling-mounted rail system, which allows the system to be shared between two operating rooms. A magnet room that is separated from the operating room via sliding radiofrequency- and sound-shielded doors allows the magnet to be used for diagnostic studies when not used in the surgical theater. The suite is designed around the IMRIS magnet and features an MR-compatible operating room table, application-specific 8-channel intraoperative radiofrequency coils, and head fixation

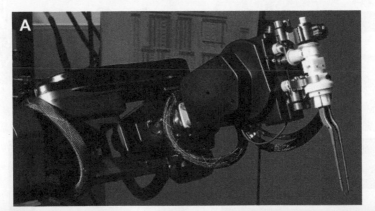

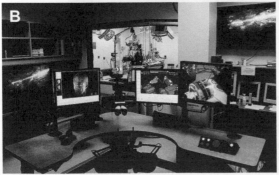
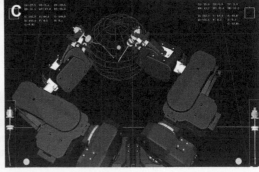

**Fig. 6.** The NeuroArm MRI-compatible neurosurgical robot. (*A*) Detailed picture of one of the NeuroArm's two operative limbs, with bipolar cautery attachment. (*B*) Command center for NeuroArm robot, where surgeon is seated and driving the movements of the robot through haptic-feedback controllers. (*C*) Real-time virtual reality display of the robot's position is delivered to the surgeon. Other virtual reality displays feature colocalization of MRI, functional MRI, and diffusion tensor imaging. (*Courtesy of* NeuroArm, Calgary, Alberta, Canada.)

devices specifically designed to fit with the IMRIS operating room table and radiofrequency coils. Nine systems have been installed worldwide, with more than 1000 surgeries performed with these systems. Twelve additional systems are currently in stages of installation. The next generation IMRIS suites will feature a 3-T magnet with capacity for biplanar angiography within the magnet room.

## FUTURE HORIZONS OF INTRAOPERATIVE MRI
### Intraoperative MRI Robotics

In the iMRI suite, manual manipulation of instruments limits the precision and repeatability of placement, particularly when surgeons have their attention divided between multiple surgical team members, image displays, and the surgical field.

As closed-bore systems predominate, the ability to manipulate tools remotely becomes increasingly important. For this reason, several groups have considered the use of instrument manipulation via robotics.[48,49] In the late 1990s, Chinzei and colleagues[50] developed one of the first MRI-compatible robotic manipulators, and the resulting positioning device was integrated into the MRT to form an MRI-guided interventional system.[51–53] Despite its revolutionary concept, this robot is designed exclusively for the original open-bore 0.5-T MRT, so its use is limited to few facilities. An MRI-compatible surgical robot suited for the new generation of closed-bore iMRI systems may offer more applicability and versatility in the neurosurgical community at large.

To enhance a surgeon's ability within the closed-bore iMRI environment, Sutherland and

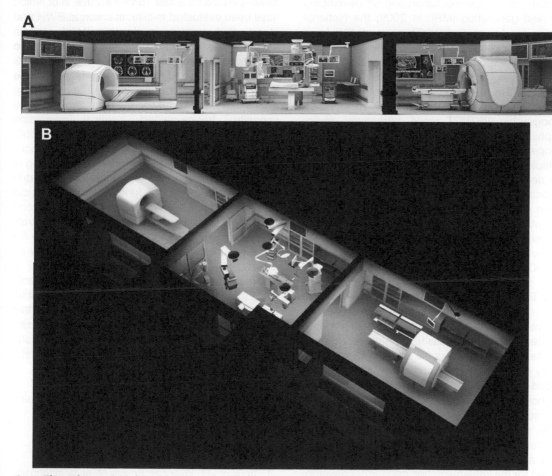

**Fig. 7.** The Advanced Multimodality Image Guided Operative (AMIGO) suite at the National Center for Image Guided Therapy, BWH and the Harvard Medical School. In AMIGO, real-time anatomic imaging modalities such as radiography and ultrasound are combined with the cross-sectional digital imaging systems of PET-CT and MRI. (*A, B*) Cross-sectional and oblique views of the three-room suite composed of a PET-CT (*left room*), state-of-the-art operating room, and 3.0T MRI (*right room*). (*Courtesy of* GE Healthcare, Wauwatosa, WI; with permission.)

colleagues[54] developed an MRI-compatible neurosurgical robot, the NeuroArm (**Fig. 6**). The robot is compact enough to function within the confines of the 70-cm bore MRI, is entirely MRI compatible, and features haptic feedback. The latter feature is a significant step in the progression of neurosurgical assistive technologies, because real-time tactile feedback is known to reduce error and increase efficiency.[49,55] Haptic data may be recorded in a real case and replayed off-line. This feature represents a powerful educational tool for neurosurgeons-in-training, allowing them to develop an understanding of tactile experience of manipulating delicate neural tissue.

## FUTURE INTRAOPERATIVE MRI SUITES

Since the first biopsy was performed in the BWH MRT in 1995, researchers, engineers, and surgeons have been collaborating on developing the next-generation iMRI. In 2009, the National Center for Image Guided Therapy at BWH will open the Advanced Multimodality Image Guided Operating (AMIGO) suite, a multimodality image-guided operating suite dedicated to intraoperative guidance (**Fig. 7**).[56] The suite will allow neurosurgeons to use 3-T MRI scans, positron emission tomographic (PET)/CT scans, ultrasound, radiographic fluoroscopy, and microscopy to update preoperative plans. The seamless unification of multiple intraoperative images promises the effective delivery of superior care for a wide range of medical conditions.

The AMIGO will be a three-room, 5700-sq-ft interventional suite with an operating room and, on opposing sides of it, a GE (Waukesha, Wisconsin) Discovery STE 64-slice PET-CT scanner and a GE 3T 750 DVMR scanner. Staff will move patients under general anesthesia via a specialized surgical table through the operating room, PET suite, and MR suite using the table's wheels or between the patient beds of the PET and MR suite on a mobile transfer tabletop. The seamless nature of patient transfer helps to address the concern over patient safety prompted by previous generations of static closed-bore iMRI systems. Other imaging devices will include ultrasound, radiographic fluoroscopes, and surgical navigation equipment. All components are designed to function in an integral manner.

As a state-of-the-art suite, the AMIGO is designed for the implementation and further development and refinement of multimodal imaging in diagnosis and therapy, such as enabling biopsies and the removal of any unwanted tissue to occur with enhanced accuracy during the same treatment session. Within the AMIGO, imaging modalities will be used in conventional and novel ways. For example, in addition to being used as it customarily is, ultrasound will be tested under research protocols within the AMIGO for its potential to monitor brain shift in real-time during neurosurgery.[56] The new understandings and techniques emerging from within the AMIGO will enable clinicians to better understand areas of interest; plan, monitor, or change treatment; navigate through a procedure or operation; and know how, where, and when to best apply a novel therapy.

## SUMMARY

In this article, we present a comprehensive framework describing the motivation, development, and evolution of contemporary iMRI in neurosurgery. We describe several key iMRI systems that have developed over the last 15 years, several of which have been evaluated in clinical cases at BWH and others that remain in developmental stages. Although the origins of iMRI can be traced to open-bore MRI at the BWH MRT, the framework for future growth and refinement will be applicable in closed-MRI systems and multimodal operating rooms that are currently on the cusp of operational capacity. Image-guided surgical navigation systems and robotics will be invaluable for applications in closed, high-field MRI magnets, particularly for applications in which real-time imaging is critical. Because targeting with submillimetric precision is required for functional neurosurgical procedures such as deep brain stimulation, gene therapy, and cell transplantation therapeutic strategies, iMRI suites will be of great importance for the future success of functional neurosurgery as a field.

The iMRI suite is a hybrid, combining elements of an interventional radiology unit, an MRI facility, and operating room. In this setting, the respective role and communication among team members (eg, surgeons, radiologists, MR technologists, nurses, anesthesiologists, computer scientists, and engineers) is of paramount importance. In the increasingly technologically driven field of medicine and science, the human factor remains the most critical.

## REFERENCES

1. Tronnier VM, Wirtz CR, Knauth M, et al. Intraoperative diagnostic and interventional magnetic resonance imaging in neurosurgery. Neurosurgery 1997;40(5):891–900.

2. Wirtz CR, Tronnier VM, Bonsanto MM, et al. Image-guided neurosurgery with intraoperative MRI:

update of frameless stereotaxy and radicality control. Stereotact Funct Neurosurg 1997;68(1–4 Pt 1):39–43.

3. Maurer CR Jr, Hill DL, Martin AJ, et al. Investigation of intraoperative brain deformation using a 1.5-T interventional MR system: preliminary results. IEEE Trans Med Imaging 1998;17(5):817–25.

4. Nimsky C, Ganslandt O, Hastreiter P, et al. Intraoperative compensation for brain shift. Surg Neurol 2001;56(6):357–64 [discussion: 64–5].

5. Ferrant M, Nabavi A, Macq B, et al. Serial registration of intraoperative MR images of the brain. Med Image Anal 2002;6(4):337–59.

6. Soza G, Grosso R, Labsik U, et al. Fast and adaptive finite element approach for modeling brain shift. Comput Aided Surg 2003;8(5):241–6.

7. Hastreiter P, Rezk-Salama C, Soza G, et al. Strategies for brain shift evaluation. Med Image Anal 2004;8(4):447–64.

8. Clatz O, Delingette H, Talos IF, et al. Robust nonrigid registration to capture brain shift from intraoperative MRI. IEEE Trans Med Imaging 2005;24(11):1417–27.

9. Berger MS, Deliganis AV, Dobbins J, et al. The effect of extent of resection on recurrence in patients with low grade cerebral hemisphere gliomas. Cancer 1994;74(6):1784–91.

10. Claus EB, Horlacher A, Hsu L, et al. Survival rates in patients with low-grade glioma after intraoperative magnetic resonance image guidance. Cancer 2005;103(6):1227–33.

11. Keles GE, Anderson B, Berger MS. The effect of extent of resection on time to tumor progression and survival in patients with glioblastoma multiforme of the cerebral hemisphere. Surg Neurol 1999;52(4):371–9.

12. Lacroix M, Abi-Said D, Fourney DR, et al. A multivariate analysis of 416 patients with glioblastoma multiforme: prognosis, extent of resection, and survival. J Neurosurg 2001;95(2):190–8.

13. Berger MS, Rostomily RC. Low grade gliomas: functional mapping resection strategies, extent of resection, and outcome. J Neurooncol 1997;34(1):85–101.

14. Fernandez-Hidalgo OA, Vanaclocha V, Vieitez JM, et al. High-dose BCNU and autologous progenitor cell transplantation given with intra-arterial cisplatinum and simultaneous radiotherapy in the treatment of high-grade gliomas: benefit for selected patients. Bone Marrow Transplant 1996;18(1):143–9.

15. Johannesen TB, Langmark F, Lote K. Progress in long-term survival in adult patients with supratentorial low-grade gliomas: a population-based study of 993 patients in whom tumors were diagnosed between 1970 and 1993. J Neurosurg 2003;99(5):854–62.

16. McGirt MJ, Chaichana KL, Gathinji M, et al. Independent association of extent of resection with

survival in patients with malignant brain astrocytoma. J Neurosurg 2008;110:156–62.

17. Sakata K, Hareyama M, Komae T, et al. Supratentorial astrocytomas and oligodendrogliomas treated in the MRI era. Jpn J Clin Oncol 2001;31(6):240–5.

18. Wirtz CR, Knauth M, Staubert A, et al. Clinical evaluation and follow-up results for intraoperative magnetic resonance imaging in neurosurgery. Neurosurgery 2000;46(5):1112–20 [discussion: 20–2].

19. Gronemeyer D, Seibel R, Erbel R, et al. Equipment configuration and procedures: preferences for interventional microtherapy. J Digit Imaging 1996;9(2):81–96.

20. Gronemeyer DH, Seibel RM, Schmidt A, et al. Two- and three-dimensional imaging for interventional MRI and CT guidance. Stud Health Technol Inform 1996;29:62–76.

21. Schenck JF, Jolesz FA, Roemer PB, et al. Superconducting open-configuration MR imaging system for image-guided therapy. Radiology 1995;195(3):805–14.

22. Alexander E 3rd, Moriarty TM, Kikinis R, et al. The present and future role of intraoperative MRI in neurosurgical procedures. Stereotact Funct Neurosurg 1997;68(1–4 Pt 1):10–7.

23. Alexander E 3rd, Moriarty TM, Kikinis R, et al. Innovations in minimalism: intraoperative MRI. Clin Neurosurg 1996;43:338–52.

24. Moriarty TM, Kikinis R, Jolesz FA, et al. Magnetic resonance imaging therapy: intraoperative MR imaging. Neurosurg Clin N Am 1996;7(2):323–31.

25. Kanal E. An overview of electromagnetic safety considerations associated with magnetic resonance imaging. Ann N Y Acad Sci 1992;649:204–24.

26. Kanal E, Borgstede JP, Barkovich AJ, et al. American College of Radiology White Paper on MR Safety: 2004 update and revisions. AJR Am J Roentgenol 2004;182(5):1111–4.

27. Kanal E, Borgstede JP, Barkovich AJ, et al. American College of Radiology White Paper on MR Safety. AJR Am J Roentgenol 2002;178(6):1335–47.

28. Kettenbach J, Kacher DF, Kanan AR, et al. Intraoperative and interventional MRI: recommendations for a safe environment. Minim Invasive Ther Allied Technol 2006;15(2):53–64.

29. Black PM, Moriarty T, Alexander E 3rd, et al. Development and implementation of intraoperative magnetic resonance imaging and its neurosurgical applications. Neurosurgery 1997;41(4):831–42 [discussion: 42–5].

30. Gering DT, Nabavi A, Kikinis R, et al. An integrated visualization system for surgical planning and guidance using image fusion and an open MR. J Magn Reson Imaging 2001;13(6):967–75.

31. Nabavi A, Black PM, Gering DT, et al. Serial intraoperative magnetic resonance imaging of brain shift. Neurosurgery 2001;48(4):787–97 [discussion: 97–8].

32. Archip N, Clatz O, Whalen S, et al. Compensation of geometric distortion effects on intraoperative magnetic resonance imaging for enhanced visualization in image-guided neurosurgery. Neurosurgery 2008;62(3 Suppl 1):209–15 [discussion: 15–6].

33. Oh DS, Black PM. A low-field intraoperative MRI system for glioma surgery: is it worthwhile? Neurosurg Clin N Am 2005;16(1):135–41.

34. Jolesz FA, Talos IF, Schwartz RB, et al. Intraoperative magnetic resonance imaging and magnetic resonance imaging-guided therapy for brain tumors. Neuroimaging Clin N Am 2002;12(4):665–83.

35. Hadani M, Spiegelman R, Feldman Z, et al. Novel, compact, intraoperative magnetic resonance imaging-guided system for conventional neurosurgical operating rooms. Neurosurgery 2001;48(4):799–807 [discussion: 9].

36. Gerlach R, du Mesnil de Rochemont R, Gasser T, et al. Feasibility of Polestar N20, an ultra-low-field intraoperative magnetic resonance imaging system in resection control of pituitary macroadenomas: lessons learned from the first 40 cases. Neurosurgery 2008;63(2):272–84 [discussion: 84–5].

37. Ntoukas V, Krishnan R, Seifert V. The new generation Polestar N20 for conventional neurosurgical operating rooms: a preliminary report. Neurosurgery 2008;62(3 Suppl 1):82–9 [discussion: 89–90].

38. Samdani AF, Schulder M, Catrambone JE, et al. Use of a compact intraoperative low-field magnetic imager in pediatric neurosurgery. Childs Nerv Syst 2005;21(2):108–13 [discussion: 14].

39. Levivier M, Wikler D, De Witte O, et al. PoleStar N-10 low-field compact intraoperative magnetic resonance imaging system with mobile radiofrequency shielding. Neurosurgery 2003;53(4):1001–6 [discussion: 7].

40. Schulder M, Sernas TJ, Carmel PW. Cranial surgery and navigation with a compact intraoperative MRI system. Acta Neurochir Suppl 2003;85:79–86.

41. Kanner AA, Vogelbaum MA, Mayberg MR, et al. Intracranial navigation by using low-field intraoperative magnetic resonance imaging: preliminary experience. J Neurosurg 2002;97(5):1115–24.

42. Salas S, Brimacombe M, Schulder M. Stereotactic accuracy of a compact intraoperative MRI system. Stereotact Funct Neurosurg 2007;85(2–3):69–74.

43. Bohinski RJ, Kokkino AK, Warnick RE, et al. Glioma resection in a shared-resource magnetic resonance operating room after optimal image-guided frameless stereotactic resection. Neurosurgery 2001;48(4):731–42 [discussion: 42–4].

44. Nimsky C, Ganslandt O, Fahlbusch R. 1.5 T: intraoperative imaging beyond standard anatomic imaging. Neurosurg Clin N Am 2005;16(1):185–200 vii.

45. Lipson AC, Gargollo PC, Black PM. Intraoperative magnetic resonance imaging: considerations for the operating room of the future. J Clin Neurosci 2001;8(4):305–10.

46. Hushek SG, Martin AJ, Steckner M, et al. MR systems for MRI-guided interventions. J Magn Reson Imaging 2008;27(2):253–66.

47. Hall WA, Truwit CL. Intraoperative MR-guided neurosurgery. J Magn Reson Imaging 2008;27(2):368–75.

48. Louw DF, Fielding T, McBeth PB, et al. Surgical robotics: a review and neurosurgical prototype development. Neurosurgery 2004;54(3):525–36 [discussion: 36–7].

49. McBeth PB, Louw DF, Rizun PR, et al. Robotics in neurosurgery. Am J Surg 2004;188(4A Suppl):68S–75S.

50. Chinzei K, Miller K. Towards MRI guided surgical manipulator. Med Sci Monit 2001;7(1):153–63.

51. Hata N, Tokuda J, Hurwitz S, et al. MRI-compatible manipulator with remote-center-of-motion control. J Magn Reson Imaging 2008;27(5):1130–8.

52. Dimaio SP, Archip N, Hata N, et al. Image-guided neurosurgery at Brigham and Women's Hospital. IEEE Eng Med Biol Mag 2006;25(5):67–73.

53. DiMaio SP, Pieper S, Chinzei K, et al. Robot-assisted needle placement in open-MRI: system architecture, integration and validation. Stud Health Technol Inform 2006;119:126–31.

54. Sutherland GR, Latour I, Greer AD. Integrating an image-guided robot with intraoperative MRI: a review of the design and construction of neuroArm. IEEE Eng Med Biol Mag 2008;27(3):59–65.

55. Rizun PR, McBeth PB, Louw DF, et al. Robot-assisted neurosurgery. Semin Laparosc Surg 2004;11(2):99–106.

56. Advanced Multimodality Image Guided Operating (AMIGO) Suite. 2008. Available at: http://www.ncigt.org/pages/AMIGO. Accessed November 2, 2008.

# Intraoperative MRI: Safety

Thomas Johnston, MD[a], Robert Moser[c], Karen Moeller, MD[a,b,c], Thomas M. Moriarty, MD[a,c,d],*

## KEYWORDS

- MRI safety • iMRI • Infection control
- Neurosurgery • Intraoperative imaging

MRI safety has been a central component of the diagnostic MRI industry. There are more than 10 million diagnostic magnetic resonance (MR) procedures performed safely each year in the United States. The American College of Radiology guidelines for diagnostic MRI facilities have ensured a very good safety record since the late 1970s. The successful incorporation of MR into the operating room requires similar adherence to strict safety guidelines and an understanding and respect for the powerful (and dangerous) physical forces of MRI. Moreover, the use of MRI during surgery creates a unique set of safety concerns for the patient including MRI interpretation and infection control challenges.

## PHYSICAL FORCES OF MRI

There are three major physical forces used in MRI that can generate a safety risk for patients and staff: the static magnetic field ($B_0$), the gradient magnetic field (dB/dt), and the radiofrequency (RF) electromagnetic field. The major risks in the MR environment related to these forces are projectiles, burns, dislodged ferromagnetic implants, and medical device malfunction or failure.

The $B_0$ is the main magnetic field of the MR scanner. It is always "on." Its primary function is the alignment of protons. There is substantial literature on the potential biophysical risks of large magnetic fields including extensive study on animals and human exposure in industrial settings.[1,2] To date, there have been no firmly established adverse effects of magnetic fields of up to 3T. The mechanical effects of $B_0$, however, are extremely dangerous. The magnetic field is highest at the magnet and decays over distance from the magnet (spatial gradient). The MR safe line is defined at 5 G (1T = 10,000 G). Thus, all MR installations have a unique gauss plot to define the area around the device (**Fig. 1**). The implication for safety is critical. Ferromagnetic objects brought within the magnetic field will be accelerated across the spatial gradient (drawn from lower to higher magnetic force) until impact at the magnet. The heavier the object, the faster the acceleration and higher the potential energy delivery to health care workers or the patient near the intraoperative MRI (iMRI) (**Fig. 2**). Diagnostic MR facility safety programs are very sensitive to the dangers of the static magnetic field. iMR centers must also recognize the dangers of rotational forces exerted on objects in the static field. All surgical tools used in iMRI must be cleared for potential ferromagnetic content. Tools with little or no ferromagnetic content can be considered "MR compatible" and used within the magnet during imaging. Other tools can be considered "MR safe" if the ferromagnetic content is too small to become projectiles in the static field, but high enough to degrade the quality and spatial accuracy of acquired images. These tools may be

[a] Department of Neurological Surgery, University of Louisville, 210 East Gray Street, Suite 1102, Louisville, KY 40202, USA
[b] Department of Pediatric Radiology, Kosair Childrens' Hospital, Division of Pediatric Neuroradiology, Louisville, KY, USA
[c] Norton Healthcare, 210 East Gray Street, Suite 1102, Louisville, KY 40202, USA
[d] Department of Neurological Surgery, Pediatric Neurosurgery, Kosair Childrens' Hospital, Louisville, KY, USA
* Corresponding author. Department of Neurologic Surgery, University of Louisville, 210 East Gray Street, Suite 1102, Louisville, KY 40202.
E-mail address: tmoriarty@niky.com (T.M. Moriarty).

Neurosurg Clin N Am 20 (2009) 147–153
doi:10.1016/j.nec.2009.04.007
1042-3680/09/$ – see front matter © 2009 Published by Elsevier Inc.

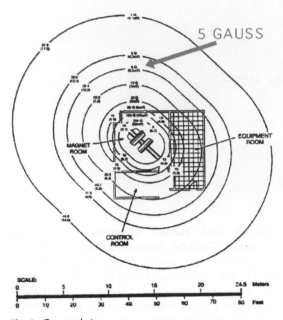

**Fig. 1.** Gauss plot.

useful during surgery, but must be respected for their likelihood of rotating within the field to align with $B_0$.

The second major physical force in MR is the dB/dt. During image acquisition, a smaller magnetic field is applied across the main field at varying angles and times to create perturbations of $B_0$. This permits the localization of protons. The safety concerns of the gradient field include the induction of voltage or current in tissues or implants (Faraday's law: changing magnetic field induces current). It has the potential to induce neural or muscular activation and create heat within tissues. It is the major source of noise in the MR environment. The gradient field can cause

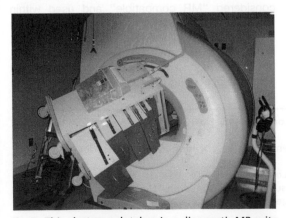

**Fig. 2.** This photograph taken in a diagnostic MR suite illustrates the risk of violating the spatial magnetic field with an anesthesia cart.

induced voltage in conductive objects (eg, pacemaker), instrument movement or failure, and spatial artifacts in the images. To limit the risks of the gradient field, all scanners are optimized to function at low dB/dt (time rate of change of gradient magnetic field<20T/s).

The third physical force in MRI is the RF electromagnetic field ($B_1$) which induces the excitation of protons. The main risk of the RF field is heating. The energy generated by $B_1$ is quantified in watts or kilograms and referred to as the specific absorption rate. It is one thousand times stronger than dB/dt and can cause burns, interfere with powered instruments (eg, anesthesia equipment), and induce currents in looped conductors (eg, a Bovie electrocautery wire). The danger of RF is addressed by limiting the specific absorption rate, avoiding looped wires near the patient or staff, and individually screening equipment for compatibility with the RF field in the ranges used for iMRI cases.

## PHYSICAL SAFETY STANDARDS

iMRI suites and their designated perioperative areas follow implemented safety guidelines and practices that were set forth by the American College of Radiology for diagnostic MRI facilities. An additional set of practices unique to those facilities involved in interventional procedures is also necessary for staff, patient, and physician safety. Standard physical safety protocols at Norton Hospital (Louisville, Kentucky) for the 0.5T "double-doughnut" General Electric Medical Systems, are referenced as general guidelines for safe surgical intervention in this article.[3–5]

## THE IMRI SUITE AND ZONE RESTRICTIONS

MRI suites are sectioned into zones based on the level of physical risk from the magnet and are designed to prevent injuries to patients, staff, and property (**Fig. 3**). A protocol for creating and maintaining four zones is now followed for such purposes. Zone I is open to all staff, patients, and the general public as a transition zone for entrance into the MRI suites' functional areas. No specific level of training is needed for staff access. zone II is the gateway from an area of no magnetic danger (zone I) to an area that may be included in the 5-G line perimeter (zones III or IV).[3,4] A potentially dangerous amount of static magnetic field is assumed to be within the 5-G line, which can cause harm to ferromagnetic substances, equipment in the area, and persons. Static magnetic fields cause objects to become missiles. Therefore, all patients are monitored in zone II and are

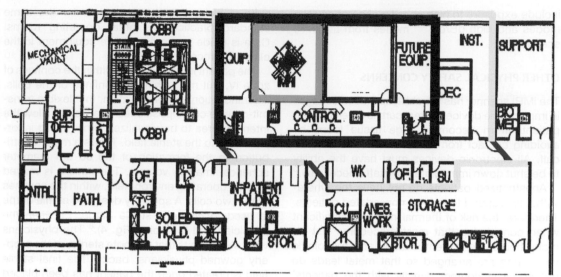

**Fig. 3.** iMRI suite at Norton Hospital with safety zones delimited by color: II, yellow; III, blue; IV, green.

checked with extensive questioning about the presence of any implantations or ferromagnetic materials. Zone III consists of a restricted area that is constantly under the supervision of MR personnel. The risk of injury from the static magnetic field in zone III is constantly present. The health of the employees and patients, along with the protection of the MR equipment, is the responsibility of the MR medical director. This responsibility could be assigned to a physician designated for the day who has the appropriate Level 2 training. Zone III typically consists of the control room or computer room and is the direct connection with zone IV, which includes the magnet and the fringe field within the 5-G line. Zone IV necessitates the strictest of compliance with safety regulations and for constant supervision of non-Level 2 personnel and patients. The 0.5T, General Electric double-doughnut iMRI protocol used at Norton Hospital uses a labeling system for all electronic devices considered for entrance into zone IV. Those devices deemed acceptable for use are labeled in green while those unacceptable for entrance into zone IV are labeled in red.[3-5]

## PERSONNEL TRAINING

iMRI-trained personnel have either Level 1 or Level 2 certification. Level 1 personnel have passed minimal safety education for work in zones I to III. This includes live or recorded lectures deemed acceptable by the MR medical director. Level 2 personnel have comprehensive training in safety and are required have direct sight of any entrance

or exit to zone IV and to all non-Level 2 personnel. The personnel are required to train in system safety, iMRI system features, and all department policies. Electrocution hazards, heating and voltage issues, high-risk object identification, and emergency response and implementation are covered under system safety training. iMRI system features training includes scanner capabilities, techniques for minimization of artifact, coil placement, stereotactic capabilities of the system, and positioning. Anesthesia monitoring and equipment are also discussed in this section of training. The department policies section includes case booking, research protocols and study implementation, and iMRI equipment compatibility testing.[3]

## IMRI EQUIPMENT COMPATIBILITY TESTING

Devices are considered safe for use in zone IV only when strict guidelines for compatibility have been met. In considering the implementation of a protocol for equipment safety and long-term functional efficacy, the departments of biomedical engineering, iMRI, and risk management have collaborated to institute a safe-equipment designation protocol. Equipment considered for testing is first given a baseline rating and allowed for non-iMRI use by the biomedical department. It is then placed one foot closer to the isocenter than its normal alignment and tested for efficacy. Then it is left in place for 1 week and retested. The device is then used in an operative case and retested. Then the device is retested in 1 month or after five operative uses. The devices are placed in a regular schedule for maintenance. The tests include exposure to high specific-absorption ratio modes and high dB/dT[AQ4] modes from the iMRI scanner.[3]

## OTHER PHYSICAL SAFETY CONCERNS

The iMRI scanner has the ability to induce voltages in implantable devices. Great care is taken to keep patients from becoming large tissue loops by avoiding contact from hand to hand, and calf to calf. All electronic devices must have the ability to be shut down immediately by staff if necessary.[3]

Anesthetized patients do not have the where-withal to respond to pain as nonsedated patients. Therefore, the risk of thermal injuries is significant when considering that most procedures last for many hours. Heart, temperature, and neurologic monitoring are arranged so that metal leads do not come in contact directly with the patients' skin. Wires are laid out so that they do not overlap or loop.[3,4]

Patients under anesthesia wear hearing protection. This is consistent with the recommendation that nonanesthetized patients should be encouraged to wear hearing protection.[3,4] Monitoring anesthetized patients in the iMRI suite has not been a problem with the 0.5T double doughnut and there are no reported instances of anesthesia-related consequences. There are also no reported instances of anesthesia-related consequences at the University of Minnesota according to Hall and colleagues.[6] Equipment for emergency resuscitation is kept outside of the 5-G line. Should the patient require emergent intervention by such devices, the patient is moved out of the 5-G radius. This has been recommended as the safest way to avoid voltage induction and missile creation.[3,4]

Instruments that are used within the 5-G line are nonferromagnetic or low iron-content steel. Titanium has proven to be an effective and safe material in the iMRI suite.[6]

## INFECTION CONTROL IN THE IMRI SUITE

The double-doughnut design of the 0.5T midfield magnet allows for 58 cm of room for each physician, up to a total working number of two at any one time.[7] Video monitors are positioned above the operating field at or above the level of the of the physicians' heads. Sterility begins with the presence of an autoclave, a decontaminator, and instrument packaging facilities within the iMRI department. Ninety-five percent of instruments used in the iMRI suite are color-coded and grouped together for cleaning and sterilization to help alleviate the mixing of MR-compatible instruments with noncompatible instruments.[3] The iMRI

suite is cleaned and prepared under the same standard practices as other operating rooms. Care is made to restrict unsafe equipment in the cleaning process.

The patient is anesthetized within the confines of zone IV, but not within the confines of the coils. After induction and preparation, the flexible trans-mit-receive coil is positioned in a way to allow the intended area to be visualized, while being incorporated into the sterile field. This is a major contribution to the formation of the 30 cm diameter spherical imaging volume. The patient is moved into the operating environment, within the confines of the two coils. A specially designed sterile drape is used to create a sterile barrier between the physician and the coils (**Fig. 4**).[8] The physicians wear sterile vests that promote sterility of the properly gowned physicians' backs. The final sterile field is created once the patient has been placed in the correct operating position within the coils, and the physician is properly gowned and the coils properly draped (**Fig. 5**). At this point, the 0.5T double-doughnut suite allows the patient to remain in place for the duration of the procedure.

Many 1.5T high-field iMRI scanners require that procedures be performed outside of the 5-G line. The sterile field is then cleared of all non-MR compatible equipment and the patient is covered with a sterile drape. This allows for a 3 to 5 minute delay of surgery intraoperatively, including a 10 to 20 second direct transit-time delay. One series of craniotomies from the University of Minnesota approximated the incidence of infection to be 2%, considered well within acceptable limits. These infections consisted of one superficial scalp infection and the delayed formation of an abscess from *Propionibacterium acnes*.[6] A multicenter, prospective study in 1997 noted an overall non-iMRI craniotomy infection rate of 6%.[9]

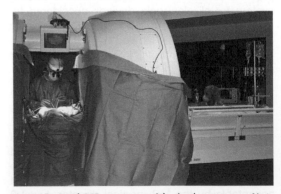

**Fig. 4.** Draped MR scanner with single surgeon. Note the sterile vest to keep the surgeon's back sterile for work within the magnet.

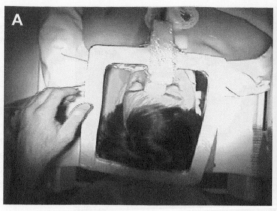
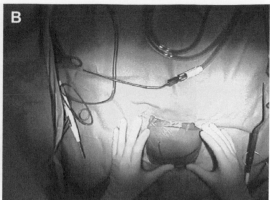

**Fig. 5.** (*A*) Application of the RF transmit-receive coil within the bore of the magnet. (*B*) Patient shaved, prepped, and draped for surgery.

The first iMRI developed and implemented was at the Brigham and Women's Hospital (Boston, Massachusetts). It was also the first 0.5T double-doughnut system, which developed in collaboration with General Electric Medical Systems and various departments at Brigham and Women's Hospital.[8] A review of the first 200 cases in the iMRI scanner at Brigham and Women's Hospital demonstrated a total infection rate of less than 1%. This included one intracranial infection after a craniotomy.[10]

## INTERPRETATION OF IMRIS

The accuracy of MRI interpretation in iMRI is of paramount safety concern. iMRI surgical procedures are guided by imaging results. Surgical decisions are made based on the image findings, and therefore, the dangerous impact of a misread is a potentially immediate threat to the safety of the patient. A close working relationship between the surgeon, radiologist, and MR technologist is the most important safety protection in this regard.

The interpretation of iMRI images presents unique challenges even for those proficient in the evaluation of routine brain MRIs. Patient positioning during an iMRI case is chosen to optimize the surgical approach to the lesion. There may be small shifts in intracranial contents in prone or decubitus positioning altering the appearance of the brain. Slice selection is determined at the surgeons request to improve visualization of the area of interest or to parallel the planned surgical course, producing oblique slice angles. Visualizing these factors before and during the operation offers a clear advantage to the surgeon over traditional stereotactic localization techniques,[10–12] while at the same time, produces images increasingly discordant from the preoperative MRI. Often

more time and consideration than expected is required to evaluate the pictures and gain a thorough understanding of the region of interest. Continued comparison to the preoperative MRI and to previous sequences obtained during the operation is the key to safe iMRI image interpretation.

Recognition of hemorrhage as it is occurring during the operation is important, but often difficult in the iMRI setting. Hyperacute hemorrhage, representing oxyhemoglobin, is isointense to brain on T1 weighted images (WI) and hyperintense on T2WI (**Fig. 6**). On T2WI, the hemorrhage may simulate saline or cerebrospinal fluid present in the surgical site, and go unrecognized. The isointense appearance of hyperacute hemorrhage on T1WI is subtle if there is no associated mass effect. Gradient echo sequences can be helpful in this scenario as the hemorrhage will demonstrate increased T2 hypointensity (blooming) distinguishing it from other fluids or tissue (**Fig. 6**).[10]

The susceptibility artifacts created by surgical tools must be respected. The actual physical size of an object will not necessarily be reflected accurately in the images. The size of the object in the image is a function of the susceptibility coefficient, MRI field strength, the image sequence used, and the orientation of phase and frequency encoding. Thus, a biopsy needle, for example, will cast a shadow in the image that is not concentric with the actual tool. The shadow may exaggerate the size and orientation of the needle by several millimeters. The accuracy of the location of the tool in the image must be confirmed in at least two image planes (**Fig. 7**). Consistency of imaging sequences, field homogeneity, and tools used will limit this potential safety problem.[13]

Interpretation of iMR images requires knowledge and skills beyond those needed for

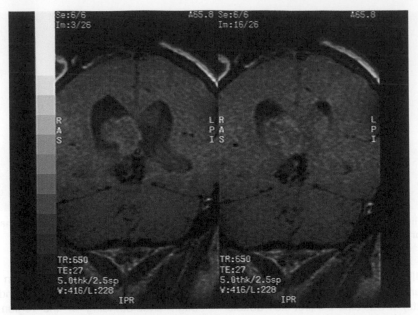

**Fig. 6.** Intraoperative hemorrhage. The image on the left shows an intraventricular tumor during surgery. The image on the right is taken later. The left lateral ventricle contains a mass of similar density as the tumor. Direct surgical inspection showed this was blood.

evaluation of routine MR images. Most of these are easily developed by the neurosurgeon and radiologist as experience is acquired. Awareness of the potential difficulties in iMR imaging along with careful comparison to preoperative studies and to previous sequences obtained during the procedure is critical. Having a technologist experienced in iMR imaging is also advantageous in optimizing image quality.

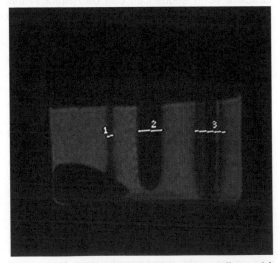

**Fig. 7.** Three experimental biopsy needles with different susceptibility coefficients imaged in an agar bath. Each has the same actual outer diameter, yet each gives a unique "size" in the MR image.

## SUMMARY

iMR scanners have great potential to assist neurosurgeons with complex procedures involving eloquent areas of the central nervous system. Respect, however, must be paid to the inherent physical dangers posed by very powerful magnetic fields, such as those within the 5-G line. Every effort is made in the realm of iMRI procedures so that current technologies help and not hinder the healing process. Knowing the imaging characteristics of iMR images and how to use effectively the information to safely carry out complex three-dimensional procedures is crucial to effective surgical management.

## REFERENCES

1. Shellock FG. Magnetic resonance procedures: health effects and safety. Boca Raton (FL): CRC Press; 2000.
2. Shellock FG, Kanal E. Magnetic resonance: bioeffects, safety, and patient management. Philadelphia: Lippincott-Raven; 1996.
3. Hushek SG, Russell L, Moser RF, et al. Safety protocols for interventional MRI. Acad Radiol 2005;12(9): 1143–8.
4. Kanal E, Borgstede JP, Barkovich AJ, et al. American College of Radiology white paper on MR safety. Am J Roentgenol 2002;178(6):1335–47.
5. Kanal E, Borgstede JP, Barkovich AJ, et al. American College of Radiology white paper on MR

safety: 2004 update and revisions. Am J Roentgenol 2004;182(5):1111–4.

6. Hall WA, Liu H, Martin AJ, et al. Safety, efficacy, and functionality of high-field strength interventional magnetic resonance imaging for neurosurgery. Neurosurgery 2000;46(3):632–42.

7. Mutchnick IS, Moriarty TM. Neurosurgical uses for intraprocedural magnetic resonance imaging. Top Magn Reson Imaging 2005;16(5):383–95.

8. Black PM, Moriarty TM, Eben A III, et al. Development and implementation of intraoperative magnetic resonance imaging and its neurosurgical applications. Neurosurgery 1997;41(4): 831–45.

9. Korinek AM. Risk factors for neurosurgical site infections after craniotomy: a prospective multicenter study of 2944 patients—the French Study Group of Neurosurgical Infections, the SEHP, the C-CLINP

Paris-Nord: service epidemiologie hygiene et prevention. Neurosurgery 1997;41(5):1073–9.

10. Schwartz RB, Hsu L, Wong TZ, et al. Intraoperative MR imaging guidance for intracranial neurosurgery: experience with the first 200 cases. Radiology 1999; 211(2):477–88.

11. Martin AJ, Hall WA, Liu H, et al. Brain tumor resection: intraoperative monitoring with high-field strength MR imaging—initial results. Radiology 2000;215(1):221–8.

12. Nimsky C, Ganslandt O, Von Keller B, et al. Intraoperative high-field strength MR imaging: implementation and experience in 200 patients. Radiology 2004;233(1):67–78.

13. Moriarty TM, Quinones-Hinojosa A, Larson PS, et al. Frameless stereotactic neurosurgery using intraoperative magnetic resonance imaging: stereotactic brain biopsy. Neurosurgery 2000;47(5):1138–46.

# Anesthesia in the Intraoperative MRI Environment

Sergio D. Bergese, MD[a],*, Erika G. Puente, MD[b]

**KEYWORDS**

- Intraoperative magnetic resonance imaging (iMRI)
- Magnetic field • MRI safety • Neurosurgery • Anesthesia

MRI is based on the magnetic resonance phenomenon and has been used for medical diagnostic imaging since 1977.[1–3] More recently, MRI technology has evolved to fulfill the needs of demanding new clinical domains. In the beginning, scanners were available only outside the operating room as a diagnostic tool. With technological advancement and incorporation of modern equipment, MRI scanners have assumed a more active role inside the operating room, providing substantial benefits as a neurosurgical tool for the treatment of neurologic diseases.

Intraoperative MRI (iMRI) can be applied in several surgical settings. It may be used for noninvasive neurologic procedures, such as the identification of eloquent brain areas. Initially, this technique was applied to assess preoperative functional brain mapping. This technology evolved into the intraoperative application of this technique, known as intraoperative functional MRI (fMRI), helping to reduce postoperative surgical morbidity of lesions in eloquent brain areas. As stated by Gasser and colleagues,[4] "fMRI is a safe and technically feasible method which allows a real-time identification of eloquent brain areas." iMRI is also used for neuronavigation during invasive neurologic procedures, providing continuous updates during surgery. Brain shift occurs after the opening of the dura and results from several factors, such as fluctuations in cerebrospinal fluid and surgical manipulation of the brain. Because the neurosurgeon has control over the MRI scanner at all times during the surgery, scans can be performed at any point deemed necessary. iMRI can be used to elucidate progressive changes in a lesion or surrounding tissue and detect complications.[5–7]

## DESIGN OF THE MRI OPERATING ROOM

The incorporation of MRI technology into the operating room requires special considerations. The size and design of the operating room, including the equipment introduced into this setting, must be MRI safe and allow adequate anesthesia monitoring and care.[8] Room size must be significantly larger than a standard operating room to allow enough space to install an MRI machine, to move the patient into and out of the MRI core, or to use a portable shield. A larger room also permits the increased number of hospital personnel involved in the patient's care to maneuver fluidly in the operating room. The magnetic field and physical structure of the unit itself creates impediments, which include difficult access to the patient for airway management and temperature control.

Another important consideration is to assure adequate distance between equipment and the location where the magnetic field is the strongest. This area is indicated by the 5 Gauss (5-G) line, within which the static magnetic field is higher than 5 G. Static magnetic field exposure to 5 G and less is considered minimal risk to bystanders. In the operating room, a clearly designated 5-G

[a] Department of Anesthesiology and Neurological Surgery, The Ohio State University Medical Center, N416 Doan Hall, 410 West 10th Avenue, Columbus, OH 43210, USA
[b] Department of Anesthesiology, The Ohio State University Medical Center, N416 Doan Hall, 410 West 10th Avenue, Columbus, OH 43210, USA
* Corresponding author.
*E-mail address:* sergio.bergese@osumc.edu (S.D. Bergese).

Neurosurg Clin N Am 20 (2009) 155–162
doi:10.1016/j.nec.2009.04.001

line and use of MR safe devices are encouraged. Because of the ferromagnetic properties of some devices, a specific distance from the magnet is required to avoid attraction of these objects. These devices should not be designated "MR safe," "MR compatible," or "intended for use in the MR environment."[1]

Two types of designs for the operating room are commonly encountered. One type of design is incorporated into the permanent construction of the operating room, most commonly used for high-field MR scanners. This arrangement requires a large infrastructural investment and fully dedicates the operating room to iMRI procedures. Typically, the operating room that contains a high-field MR scanner is entirely shielded, including the walls, ceiling, and floor. Another type of design is a mobile arrangement that can be transported into and out of the operating room as needed. The mobile design is used with most models of low-field MR scanners, such as the PoleStar N20 (Medtronic Navigation, Louisville, Colorado) at our center, which requires the use of a portable Faraday cage (**Fig. 1**). When the magnet is not in use, it is usually stored in a shielded cage. When the shield is collapsed, it takes the shape of an accordion. This closed-shield accordion consumes a relatively small amount of space against the wall when not in use. The only permanent infrastructural requirement is a floor shield under the operating room table that forms the bottom of the Faraday cage. With this arrangement the operating room is available for conventional procedures and iMRI procedures, thus providing better use of the resources.

## SET-UP TIME

For traditional neurosurgical procedures, approximate set-up time from intubation to incision can

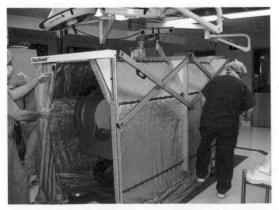

**Fig. 1.** Faraday portable shielding system being extended.

range from 0.5 to 3 hours.[5] Organization of the operating room and set-up of the patient must be meticulous because of the difficulties encountered with patient manipulation once the procedure has begun. Similar challenges may be related to patient positioning, especially in lateral and prone positions, because of a lack of armrests attached to the operating table. Another challenge involves adding extension sets to the intravenous (IV) tubing, ventilator tubing, oxygen probe, end tidal $CO_2$ monitor and ECG leads. The extension lines must be properly arranged, color-coded, and positioned along the patient's body to extend caudally. The extension lines must exit through a small outlet at the base of the Faraday cage. To eliminate part of the lengthy set-up routine for the anesthesiologist, anesthesia technicians come in before the surgery and prepare the room for this specific situation. A case series presented by Barua and colleagues[5] shows that the total set-up time continues to decrease as the anesthesiologist becomes more familiar with the process. The iMRI learning curve shows how set-up time decreased over a 21-month period (**Fig. 2**). This downward trend in the figure demonstrates how the set-up time decreases with the anesthesiologist's increasing familiarity and experience with the process.

## INTRAOPERATIVE MRI MONITORING: PATIENT AND EQUIPMENT

According to the standards for basic anesthetic monitoring, approved by the American Society of Anesthesiologists (ASA)[9] House of Delegates on October 21, 1986, and last amended on October 25, 2005:

*Every patient receiving anesthesia shall have the electrocardiogram continuously displayed from the beginning of anesthesia until preparing to leave the anesthetizing location; every patient receiving anesthesia shall have arterial blood pressure and heart rate determined and evaluated at least every five minutes; and every patient receiving general anesthesia shall have, in addition to the above, circulatory function continually evaluated by at least one of the following: palpation of a pulse, auscultation of heart sounds, monitoring of a tracing of intra-arterial pressure, ultrasound peripheral pulse monitoring, or pulse plethysmography or pulse oximetry.*

The introduction of a magnetic field into the operating room environment requires modification of equipment that is able to comply with ASA monitoring standards. These standards specifically

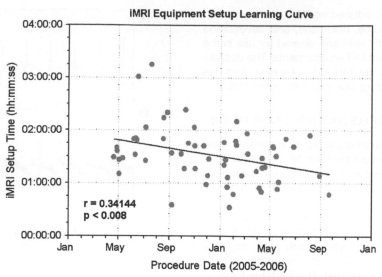

**Fig. 2.** Learning curve demonstrating decrease of set-up time with increased training of staff for 62 successful iMRI procedures over a 21-month period at the Department of Anesthesiology at the Ohio State University Medical Center (Barua et al).

require uninterrupted evaluation of the patient's oxygenation, ventilation, circulation, and temperature. Even with portable MRI scanners, the patient is confined within the bore, away from the direct supervision of the anesthesiologist for the duration of the scan. During this time, it is crucial to maintain compliance with ASA guidelines by assuring continuous ventilatory supports, inhalation anesthetics, IV drug or contrast media infusions, and patient warming (**Fig. 3**).

There are general restrictions and perils that may present in an operating room setting because of the MRI technology involving the monitoring equipment, anesthesia machine, and infusion

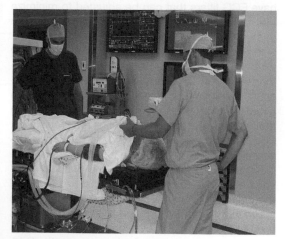

**Fig. 3.** Anesthesiologist positioning patient in the iMRI. Example of dead space in extended anesthesia circuit.

devices. The source of the electromagnetic force attracts any ferromagnetic object or instrument, such as glasses, pens, stethoscopes, scissors, IV poles, gas cylinders, laryngoscopes, and anesthesia machines. This ferromagnetic attraction poses potential injury to patients or staff in the operating room.[10]

Several monitors exist that are designed for conditional use in a magnetic resonance environment. These monitors are commonly used in MRI suites for patients undergoing managed anesthesia care or general anesthesia; however, they have not been fully tested for the complexity of neurosurgical procedures in the intraoperative MRI setting. The general design criterion in these monitors is to eliminate conductors that carry electrical signals for monitoring physiologic parameters of the patient. These conductors can function as receiving antenna on which the pulsating electrical and magnetic energy can induce spurious electric noise (EN) that distorts and corrupts the physiologic waveforms displayed on the monitor. The two general approaches currently used to achieve this criterion are the use of fiber optics and wireless technology. When metal objects and electronic monitors are introduced into the MR environment, they may interact with the images produced by the MRI scanner by reflecting or generating radiofrequency (RF) waves. These may result in distorted MR images that are unreliable for diagnostic purposes.[8]

There is negligible ferromagnetic material in vaporizers and mechanical ventilators, and with the exception of desflurane, these devices behave properly when introduced into MR environments.[8] Isoflurane, enflurane, halothane, and sevoflurane vaporizers are MR safe and cleared for use in the low- and high-field MR environments. The desflurane vaporizer is not MR safe, however, and has not been cleared for use in MR environments.

## IMPLICATIONS OF ELECTRIC NOISE GENERATION

Essentially all electronic devices in the operating room are microprocessor-based. These devices can emit spurious low-energy EN in the megahertz or gigahertz region of the RF spectrum that can interfere with the operation of other electrical equipment, including an electrically sensitive iMRI system. Devices including, but not limited to, infusion pumps, plasma and LCD displays, physiologic monitors, and computers have a measurable EN footprint. The portable Faraday cage used in low-field iMRI operating suites is designed to minimize the impact of this low-energy EN on the iMRI system. The shield encloses the patient, the magnet, the magnetic gradients, and the iMRI receiving antenna and prevents most of the spurious EN from interfering with the iMRI scan. The shield preserves the integrity of the constructed image. The manufacturers of the iMRI systems have EN algorithms to measure spurious noise to ascertain that the EN is within tolerable limits for a quality image.

One of the largest challenges for the anesthesiologist is coping with the high-energy iMRI-generated EN. An iMRI system, by design and function, generates pulsating high-energy RF signals and pulsating magnetic field gradients to capture a useful anatomic image.[11] The RF generator operates in the megahertz region of the RF spectrum and, by itself, can emit EN in the form of electromagnetic energy that can interfere with the operation of electronic patient monitors. The RF signal and the magnetic gradients of an iMRI system are pulsed during a scan at a frequency dependent on the specific imaging pulse sequence type and the parameters used. The sequences used for iMRI typically apply gradient and RF pulses at rates less than 100 Hz.[2] These high-energy pulsations can generate a significant second EN component in the frequency bandwidth of most monitored physiologic signals. The most vulnerable signal is the ECG. **Fig. 4** shows the effect of these pulsations during a scan with a 0.15 T low-field iMRI system using a conditionally compatible iMRI monitor. It can be seen that the relatively high-energy noise in the ECG produced by the pulsating magnetic field gradients has a dramatic effect on the ECG baseline signal and can mask virtually all

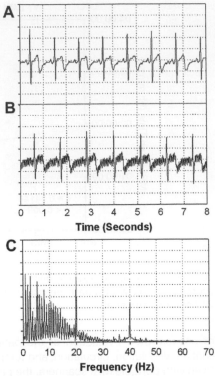

**Fig. 4.** The effect of noise produced by a 0.15 T iMRI T1 3.5-minute 4-mm scan on the ECG waveform. (*A*) Lead II ECG tracing before an iMRI scan. (*B*) ECG tracing during the scan showing the noise induced on the ECG from the magnetic gradient pulsations. (*C*) Frequency domain representation (using fast Fourier transform analysis) of the signal in b. Noise appears as a high-energy narrow band signal centered at 20 Hz and producing a 40-Hz harmonic.

details of the ECG waveform. Most monitors have ECG filters that can be adjusted to minimize the noise while maintaining as much of the rhythm information as possible.[12]

In the high-field iMRI environment, particularly when whole-body or upper-body scans are performed, the ECG is also affected by a phenomenon called hydromagnetics that describes the behavior of a fluid (in this case blood flow) in the presence of an electric or a magnetic field. The blood flow generates voltages across the vessels, which distort the ECG signal. The distortion is proportional to the velocity and volume of the blood through the vessels and the orientation of the vessel in relation to the magnetic field. A common distortion seen in the ECG is generated by blood flow in the aortic arch and ascending aorta in a magnetic field, which presents as an increase in the T-wave amplitude.[13]

## ORCHESTRATING THE INTRAOPERATIVE MRI ENVIRONMENT: AN ANESTHESIOLOGIST'S PERSPECTIVE

Introducing the MRI technology into the operating room setting presents a new challenge in a trans-disciplinary environment.[14] The anesthesiologist orchestrates safety promotion by minimizing or eliminating iMRI-associated accidents, while assuring optimal patient vigilance and monitoring. Direct patient observation may be compromised by acoustic noise, darkened environment, obstructed line of sight, and distractions. Patient safety may be compromised by medical or health-related risks, equipment-related risks, and procedure-related risks. The anesthesiologist is dually responsible for identifying functional limitations and patient risks associated with the iMRI technology.

Accounting for these limitations and risks, the anesthesiologist must conduct a thorough preoperative assessment. The anesthesiologist requires training and knowledge on complications specific to the MR environment that may confound on the patient's medical history. The anesthesiologist must perform an MRI compatibility preoperative examination. This examination should explore history of acquired or implanted metallic devices, such as cerebrovascular clips, cochlear implants, cardiac pacemakers, intravascular wires, stents, bullets, extensive tattoos, or permanent eye make-up.[15] These devices may be ferromagnetic and lead to displacement or dislodgment. Surgical clips that contain mostly nickel are not considered dangerous.[8] Patients who have braces or dentures may generate artifacts that may significantly degrade iMRI images. The heating of metallic implants can lead to severe burns, and when encountered, the patient should be immediately evacuated from the MR environment. When selecting devices for MR environment set-ups, it is necessary to verify the compatibility of the selected device with the particular scanner that will be used (**Fig. 5**).

## ECG

The following recommendations should be followed to reduce artifacts in the ECG reading. The preferred electrodes and cables should be MR safe and contain minimal metal components. While the scanner generates an image, the magnet produces EN that disables the ECG waveform monitor from producing quality readings for diagnosing cardiac arrhythmias or ischemia. In a standard MRI suite during a scan, the precordial leads are purposefully placed closer together to avoid

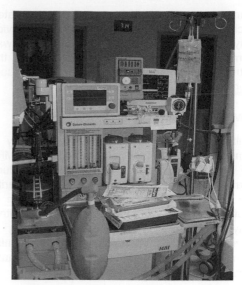

**Fig. 5.** Example of MR-safe anesthesia machine and vaporizers.

distortion generated in the ECG reading by the aortic blood flow. In contrast, in an iMRI setting where the duration of the scanning period is comparatively smaller than the duration of the entire surgical procedure, the author recommends the use of the standard distribution of precordial leads. This distribution allows better monitoring of the patient throughout the surgical procedure, even though the readings are expected to be affected by noise during scanning periods; this results in an increased amount of time for the anesthesiologist to access an ECG reading that offers a higher sensitivity for the detection of cardiac ischemia or infarction. During the time when the patient is being imaged or is enclosed in the shield, the anesthesiologist must rely entirely on indirect electronic patient monitoring. The anesthesiologist must be trained to adjust the electronic filters on the ECG monitor to achieve the most noise-free view of the ECG waveform during a scanning procedure that may last as long as 13 minutes. If a cardiac event is suspected during the procedure, the patient should be removed from the high-field MR operating room for accurate monitoring. If a similar situation occurs in a low-field MR setting, the magnet can be removed from the operative location and returned to the storage cage. At this point standard monitoring procedures and treatment may be reinitiated.

## BLOOD PRESSURE

Standard blood pressure monitoring techniques may be used with minimal adaptations. A mercury manometer, sphygmomanometer, or automated oscillometric blood pressure recording device may still be used as long as they are kept away from the scanner.[8,16] For major craniotomies, the author recommends invasive blood pressure monitoring through the use of an arterial line.

## TEMPERATURE CONTROL

Multiple factors may contribute to difficulty in temperature control for patients undergoing MRI. RF waves emitted from the magnet may produce heat and increase body temperature. Contrarily, the cold temperatures required in the room to protect against overheating of the computers may decrease body temperature. Heating of devices used in the operating room, such as pulse oximeters and temperature probes, may cause local burn injuries.[16]

## VENTILATION AND OXYGENATION

During the time that the patient is within the scanner, it may be difficult to properly visualize clinical signs of ventilation, such as chest movements, breath sounds, and reservoir bag fluctuation. When the patient is not in view of the anesthesiologist, it is impossible to identify signs of apnea or cyanosis. Because of the loud noise generated by the magnet, it may also be difficult to assess breath sounds through auscultation. MR-safe pulse oximeters are available for use in MR environments to measure oxygen saturation. Anesthesiologists may benefit by using an end-tidal $CO_2$ monitor with elongated sampling tube in anesthetized patients.

## ACOUSTIC NOISE

Another safety consideration for high-field MR environments is the acoustic noise generated from the MR machine during a scan, which can exceed 100 dB. An effective barrier against patient and operator injury from this sound is the use of foam earplugs. It is important that the use of earplugs by iMRI staff does not interfere with the ability to hear physician commands or respond to emergencies. In low-field MR environments, patients and staff may benefit from the use of earplugs during the duration of the scan, although this may not be necessary for the remainder of the surgical procedure.

## GENERAL ANESTHESIA CONSIDERATIONS

After an MR safe–oriented preoperative assessment and addressing monitoring and patient positioning, the patient may undergo general anesthesia. General anesthesia requires an extended anesthetic circuit for ventilation maintenance and drug administration because the patient is located farther from the anesthesia machine than in traditional operating room settings. Dead space creates a time delay before the volatile anesthetic and drugs are administered and when expected effects can be observed (**Fig. 6**). A combination of IV anesthetic with volatile agents is preferred. Volatile anesthetics provide practicality and reliability because of the delivery system. IV agents help to reduce the amount of inhalation agents while helping to decrease brain flow and providing a steadier anesthetic technique. In the author's experience with low-field MR settings, the use of desflurane is preferred over other agents because of its pharmacokinetic properties. The preferential IV anesthetic agents for the management of neurosurgeries are remifentanil and dexmedetomidine.[17]

Desflurane may decrease the need for diagnostic and therapeutic interventions and minimize respiratory complications. The pharmacokinetics of desflurane provide a rapid return of consciousness thus allowing prompt neurologic examination. Desflurane provides better control and stability of hemodynamics, decreasing hypertension in an effort to preface the complication of bleeding. Additionally, desflurane may reduce coughing and postoperative nausea and vomiting, which could indirectly lead to an increase in vascular pressure.[18–21]

Remifentanil hydrochloride is a member of the selective μ opioid receptor agonist family. Remifentanil has an action onset of approximately 1 minute, quickly achieving a steady state. It is rapidly metabolized by nonspecific blood and tissue esterases into a clinically inactive metabolite. Remifentanil is

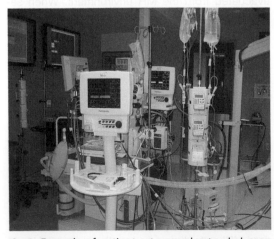

**Fig. 6.** Example of patient set-up and extended anesthesia circuit.

easily titrated because of a half-life ranging from 3 to 10 minutes. Neurosurgical anesthesiologists should consider remifentanil because it provides a better state of consciousness after discontinuation of the infusion. Remifentanil is an advantage when used in neurosurgery because it is known to decrease cerebral blood flow and reduce intracranial pressure.

Dexmedetomidine belongs to the $\alpha_2$-adrenergic receptor antagonist family and is preferred for the sympatholytic, analgesic, and sedative properties.[22] Dexmedetomidine has an action mechanism that reduces sympathetic outflow by decreasing the volume of norepinephrine released in the central nervous system. Dexmedetomidine is particularly advantageous for use in neurosurgical patients to facilitate cooperative sedation when neurologic responses must be assessed during surgery. Other properties include increased affinity for pain receptors, cardiovascular stability, reduction in anesthetic requirements, and decreased respiratory depression. Dexmedetomidine is known to maintain a more stable intracranial pressure, show better congruity with neurophysiologic monitoring, and grant superior neuroprotection. Additionally, it seems to lower cerebral blood flow generated by cerebrovascular vasoconstriction.[17]

Dexmedetomidine in combination with remifentanil decreases the required minimal alveolar concentration (MAC) levels to maintain adequate depth of anesthesia compared with the standard MAC levels.[10,22] In addition, hemodynamic stability is achieved without experiencing hypotension or bradycardia. Ultimately, the study conducted by Pangrazzi and colleagues[23] demonstrated that a more physiologic blood pressure range and lower systolic blood pressures were achieved by subjects who received dexmedetomidine versus subjects who did not.

## CONTRAST AGENT SAFETY: GADOLINIUM

Gadolinium-based contrast agents are approved by the U.S. Food and Drug Administration (FDA) for use in MRI. Even so, postmarketing reports indicate that gadolinium-based contrast has demonstrated a higher incidence in patient's developing a progressive and debilitating or fatal disease called nephrogenic systemic fibrosis (NSF). This condition is particularly exacerbated in patients who have a medical history of acute or chronic severe renal insufficiency.

For this reason, the FDA has instructed that the package inserts of all gadolinium-based agents should update the warning section and include a "Boxed Warning" indicating the increased risk

for NSF in patients who meet the following medical conditions:

> Acute or chronic severe renal insufficiency (glomerular filtration rate <30 mL/min/1.73 m$^2$), or
> Acute renal insufficiency of any severity due to the hepatorenal syndrome or in the perioperative liver transplantation period.[25]

In renal-compromised patients, the use of gadolinium-based contrast should be avoided unless the diagnostic information expected from the contrast MRI outweighs the risk of the procedure. It is necessary for the anesthesiologist to be aware of this warning and to screen all patients for renal dysfunction by obtaining the patient's medical history and reviewing laboratory test results during the preoperative evaluation. As always, the author recommends administering appropriate contrast doses and allowing sufficient time for elimination of the agent before readministration.[24]

## SUMMARY

There are multiple factors to consider when preparing a procedure to conform within an MR environment, including ensuring that the patient and equipment is MR safe before being introduced into this setting to maximize safety efforts. The anesthesiologist's role in the operating room is crucial when orchestrating the different aspects involved in a safe and successful experience for the patient and staff. It is mandatory to implement a system that reflects the involvement of multiple disciplines to ensure the highest level of delivered patient care. The use of the iMRI technology has provided revolutionary tools for the new generation of medical practice. iMRI is a dynamic innovation that has yet to reach its full potential.

## ACKNOWLEDGMENTS

The authors thank Roger Dzwonczyk and Kelly Rosborough.

## REFERENCES

1. Magnetic Resonance Imaging (MRI). Technology InformationPortal. 2008. Available at: http://www.mr-tip.com/serv1.php?type=welcome. Accessed November 15, 2008.
2. CIGNA. Magnetic Resonance Imaging (MRI), Low-Field. CIGNA Healthcare Coverage Position [coverage position number: 0444] n.p. CIGNA 2008. p. 1–21.
3. Barash PG, Cullen BF, Stoelting RK. Anesthesia for Nonoperative Locations. In: Barash PG, Cullen BF, Stoelting RK, editors. Clinical Anesthesia. 3rd edition.

Philadelphia: Lippincott-Raven Publishers; 1997. p. 1240–1.

4. Gasser T, Ganslandt O, Sandalcoglu E, et al. Intraoperative functional MRI: Implementation and preliminary experience. Neuroimage 2005;26: 685–93.

5. Barua E, Johnston J, Dzwonczyk R, et al. Anesthesia for brain tumors using intraoperative magnetic resonance imaging (iMRI) with the Polestar N-20 System: experience and challenges. J Clin Anesth; in press.

6. Nabavi A, Black PML, Gering DT, et al. Serial Intraoperative MR Imaging of Brain Shift. Neurosurgery 2001;48:787–98.

7. Hirschl R, Wilson J, Miller B, et al. The predictive value of low-field strength magnetic resonance imaging for intraoperative residual tumor detection. J Neurosurg 2009; in press.

8. Longnecker DE, Tinker JH, Morgan GE Jr. Anesthesia for Non Surgical Procedures. In: Longnecker DE, Tinker JH, Morgan GE Jr, editors. Principles and Practice of Anesthesiology 2nd edition. St. Louis: Mosby, Inc; 1998. p. 2287–94.

9. American Society of Anesthesiologists (ASA) Standards for Basic Anesthetic Monitoring. ASA Standards, Guidelines and Statements. Available at: www. ASAhq.org/publicationsAndServices/standards/ 02.pdf#2. Accessed November 15, 2008.

10. Mackenzie RA, Southron PA, Stensrud PE. Anesthesia at Remote Locations. In: Miller RD, editor. Anesthesia. 5th edition. Philadelphia: Churchill Livingstone; 2000. p. 2241–69.

11. Webster JG. Medical Imaging Systems, . Medical Instrumentation: Application and Design. 3rd edition. USA: John Wiley & Sons, Inc; 1998. 518–76.

12. Dzwonczyk R, Fujii J, Simonetti O, et al. Electrical Noise in the Intraoperative Magnetic Resonance Imaging Setting. Anesthesia & Analgesia 2009;108: 181–6.

13. Nijm G, Swiryn S, Larson A, et al. Extraction of the magnetohydrodynamic blood flow potential from the surface electrocardiogram in magnetic resonance imaging. Medical and Biological Engineering and Computing 2008;46:729–33.

14. Berkenstadt H, Perel A, Ram Z, et al. Anesthesia for Magnetic Resonance Guided Neurosurgery. Journal of Neurosurgical Anesthesiology 2001;13(2): 158–62.

15. Gooden C, Dilos B. Anesthesia for Magnetic Resonance Imaging. Curr Opin Anaesthesiol 2004; 17(4):339–42.

16. Bell C. Anesthesia in the MRI Suite. GASNet Inc. Available at: http://clinicalwindow.net/dl/cw_paper_ mri_bell.pdf. Accessed November 20, 2008.

17. Bekker A, Sturaitis M. Dexmedetomidine for Neurological Surgery. Operative Neurosurgery 2005;57: ONS1–ONS10.

18. Ghouri AF, Bodner M, White PF. Recovery profile after desflurane-nitrous oxide versus isoflurane-nitrous oxide in outpatients. Anesthesiology 1991; 74(3):419–24.

19. Nathanson MH, Fredman B, Smith I, et al. Sevoflurane versus desflurane for outpatient anesthesia: a comparison of maintenance and recovery profiles. Anesthesia and Analgesia 1995;81(6):1186–90.

20. Parr SM, Robinson BJ, Glover PW, et al. Sevoflurane versus desflurane for outpatient anesthesia: a comparison of maintenance and recovery profiles. Anesthesia Intensive Care 1991;19(3):369–72.

21. Boisson-Bertrand D, Laxenaire MC, Lapeyre G. Emergence and Recovery from Desflurane or Isoflurane Prolonged Anaesthesia for Acoustic Neuroma Surgical Procedures [abstract A. 464]. Br J Anaesth 1998;80(suppl1):136.

22. Bergese SD, Khabiri B, Roberts WD, et al. Case Report: Dexmedetomidine for conscious sedation in difficult awake fiberoptic intubation cases. J Clin Anesth 2007;19:141–4.

23. Pangrazzi G, Uhler J, Vaadyala P, et al. Dexmedetomidine Lowers the Concentration of Anesthetic Required during Craniotomies below MAC [Abstract A1461]. In: ASA Annual Meeting Abstracts. Orlando: 2008. Found at http://www.asaabstracts. com/strands/asaabstracts/abstract.htm;jsessionid= 8C54A6AE9853D45781F15460851F3CC4?year= 2008&index=7&absnum=1977. Accessed November 4, 2008.

24. Kanal E, Barkovich AJ, Bell C, et al. The Practice of Radiology. Original Research. ACR Guidance Document for Safe MR Practices: 2007. American Journal of Roentgenology 2007;188:1447–74.

25. MAGNEVIST (gadopentetate dimeglumine) injection. Bayer HealthCare Pharmaceuticals Inc. Available at: http://dailymed.nlm.nih.gov/dailymed/ drugInfo.cfm?id=8429. Accessed November 15, 2008.

# Intraoperative MRI with 1.5 Tesla in Neurosurgery

Arya Nabavi, MD*, Lutz Dörner, MD, Andreas M. Stark, MD,
H. Maximilian Mehdorn, MD, PhD

**KEYWORDS**

- Intraoperative MRI • Neurosurgery • Brain tumor
- Brain shift • Updated neuronavigation • Open magnet

High-field (1.5 T) MRI has been successfully integrated into the operating theater. State-of-the-art microneurosurgical equipment and computer-assisted navigation are merged with the intraoperative MRI (iMRI) to form a comprehensive unit. iMRI was once deemed an inaccessible vision. However, after low- and midfield systems provided a "proof of concept,"[1–5] high-field magnets were soon integrated into the operating room (OR).[6,7] Since the first reports, more centers have taken steps toward using high-field iMRI. Whereas high-field iMRI provides superior image quality in a variety of applicable sequences,[8] it also presents new challenges. The authors report on their implementation of 1.5 T high-field iMRI in an integrated magnetic resonance operating room (MR-OR), illustrate their approach and application.

## COMMON FEATURES OF 1.5 TESLA INTRAOPERATIVE MRI SYSTEMS

The 1.5T magnets used for iMRI are essentially the same as those used for diagnostic applications. Because of this, all sequences used for diagnostics can be used intraoperatively. The standard structural imaging used during iMRI are T1 (gadolinium enhanced or non-enhanced), T2, and fluid attenuated inversion recovery (FLAIR). To address specific issues, diffusion tensor imaging (DTI), spectroscopy, diffusion-weighted images, heme sequences, and MR-angiography have been reported.[6,7,9–11]

The suites require shielding to reduce interference by radio frequency (RF) noise. The surgical and imaging areas are separated by the 5-G line for safety reasons. Ceiling-mounted flat panel monitors provide visualization of preoperative and intraoperative imaging data, and real-time views of the surgical field.

Most MR-ORs have been equipped with navigation systems,[12] which provide the link for updated navigation. At our institution, the ceiling-mounted monitors and detection camera are connected to the computer in the separate MR console room. Navigation is used for both initial planning and throughout surgery, with imaging data updated at the surgeon's discretion, to guide the resection and compensate for intraoperative deformations.[13,14]

Time restraints are a major consideration for iMRI. To finish surgery in a timely fashion, it is necessary to obtain the maximum of imaging information with the shortest possible imaging time. Potential advances lie in imaging and coil technology. The most commonly used "parallel imaging" in diagnostics can be employed intraoperatively as well, with the appropriate coil technology.[15] Modified coil designs, combined with the head fixation and with fiducials for automated registration, and flexible coils placed around the carbon fiber head-fixation have been implemented.[6,15]

Imaging technology may yield other potential time savers. Different tissue characteristics may

The MRI was acquired through a grant from the German Federal Government (BMBF 01 EZ 0103).
Department of Neurosurgery, University Hospital Schleswig-Holstein, Campus Kiel, Schittenhelmstr 10, 24105 Kiel, Germany
* Corresponding author.
*E-mail address:* nabavia@nch.uni-kiel.de (A. Nabavi).

be captured simultaneously and subsequently extracted from this common data set: T1-weighted images (WI) and double echo from a single acquisition.[16] This so-called "synthetic imaging" or similar techniques may provide significant reduction in imaging time.

## DISTINCT FEATURES OF 1.5 TESLA IMRI SYSTEMS

Since the areas for imaging and actual surgery are separate in many clinical circumstances using iMRI, either the patient is transferred to the MRI, or the MRI is brought to the patient.

### Magnetic Resonance-to-Patient Transport

The first installation of a mobile MRI was in Calgary, Canada.[6] In this scenario, the magnet is brought into the OR on ceiling mounted rails ("overhead crane technology"). It usually resides in a shielded room next to the OR. This arrangement allows for surgery with conventional surgical instruments. The operating table is MR-compatible and hydraulic-controlled, permitting customary patient positioning. For scanning, ferromagnetic instruments are removed from within the 5-G line of the magnet's approach path and final position. The coils and the head holder are combined into a single unit. The RF coil system can be separated into a bottom half and a top half. The top half can be removed during surgery and replaced in a sterile fashion for iMRI.

### Patient-to-Magnetic Resonance Transfer

#### The Minnesota (United States) or Kiel (Germany) solution

The first installation of a stationary, short bore high-field MRI within a neurosurgical suite was in Minneapolis, Minnesota.[7,9] In this particular scenario, a modified angiography-MRI unit originally developed to allow conventional angiographies or interventions is located outside the 5-G line. The angiography table mount is in continuity with the MRI-bore, and the patient is transferred on a mobile tabletop. For surgery, the table can be turned 35° from the MR-bore long axis, placing the patient's head well outside the 5-G line, permitting the use of ferromagnetic instruments. Table mobility permits height regulation, and tilting of the head holder. For imaging, the table is returned to the original position, reconnected to the table mount, and the patient is slid on the tabletop into the bore. Ferromagnetic material has to be removed. As a special feature of this design, the table can extend beyond the rear of the MRI. For surgery in the "back of the magnet," MR-compatible instruments are necessary, since

this surgical area lies within the 5-G line. This design is the only one with a short bore and wide entrance to the tunnel, which allows access to the patient for real-time imaging. At our institution, we have a modified installation of this prototype (see later discussion).

### The Erlangen (Germany) solution

The second possibility for integrating an MRI into an OR differs from the aforementioned basically by the arrangement of the surgical table.[11,15]

The surgical table is rotated around its base 160° away from the MR-axis, placing the patient's head just inside the 5-G line (called the "fringe field"). The specially designed MR-table allows modifying the height and the lateral and axial tilt. The coils are integrated into the rigid headholder, providing "parallel imaging" capabilities. The separable top portion is removed during surgery, and replaced for imaging.

### Kiel set-up

We realized a fully integrated MRI-OR at our institution in 2005. At the core of this OR is a short-bore, 1.5T Scanner (Philips Intera, Philips Medical Systems, Best, Netherlands).

The OR can be divided into areas within, on the border (fringe field), and outside the 5-G line. Our primary surgical area for microneurosurgery is outside of the 5-G line, using ferromagnetic tools and equipment. This area is equipped with a ceiling-mounted navigation system (BrainLab VectorVision), which allows conventional neuronavigation with preoperative and updated navigation with intraoperatively acquired images (**Fig. 1**A). The patient is transferred from the primary microneurosurgical operating site to the scanner (imaging site) using a pivotal angiography table (modified Angio DIAGNOS 5 Syncra Tilt Patient Support, Philips Medical Systems, Best, Netherlands), which connects to the MRI (**Fig. 1**B, C). For this transfer, the surgical site is draped. MRI images are obtained and loaded into our navigation system while the patient is transferred back to the surgical area. Thus, the neuronavigation system can be used for accurate navigation with renewed image data.

Secondary surgical sites (**Fig. 2**) are in the fringe field and "behind" the MRI. Surgery in the fringe field (see **Fig. 2**A) permits the use of ferromagnetic instruments and techniques as in our primary surgical area. It is slightly more restricted since neither table height, nor angulation can be altered.

The area behind the MRI (see **Fig. 2**B, C) is within the magnetic field. The magnetic pull of the field is palpable when ferromagnetic instruments are used, but the pull is not strong enough

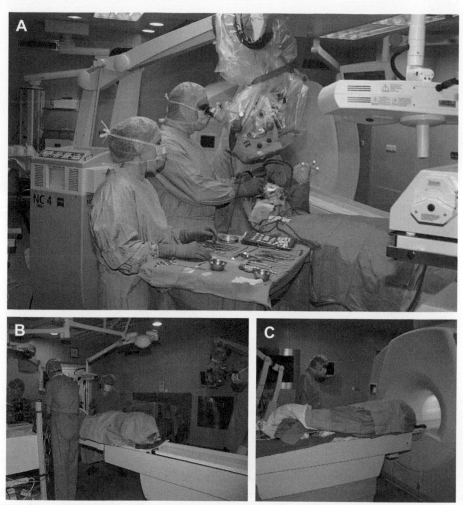

**Fig. 1.** Primary surgical area and transfer to MRI for imaging. (*A*) Routine set-up. The table is rotated 35° away from the MRI axis. The surgical site with the microscope is outside of the 5-G line. The scrub nurse and her set-up are on the patient's side, away from the MRI. Ferromagnetic instruments (standard set is on the table, same as conventional OR) are kept away from the MRI. Any further instruments are brought in directly to the nurse, thus keeping helpers and traffic away from the MRI. The camera system of the navigation system with the monitor (out of view) is suspended from the ceiling. Bipolar and ultrasonic aspirators are in front of the nurse. (*B, C*) The patient's transfer from the primary surgical site to the scanner. The operating site is draped in a sterile fashion, and additional draping placed on top. The floating tabletop is brought in line with the MRI axis. Then the patient is pushed toward the scanner, where positioning is automated.

to hamper their use. Bipolar and ultrasonic aspirator and conventional scalpel and sutures can be used here. At present, OR microscopes do not function this far within the 5-G line. This site permits rapid transfer of the patient into the scanner, even without additional draping. Although transfer from the primary surgical site is not lengthy, from this site it is even shorter. However since this area is without a microscope, we limit its use to cases where repeated scanning is probable. After the first scan, we decide whether to proceed with surgery outside the 5-G line, or behind the MRI.

Since September, 2005, we have operated on 350 patients using intraoperative imaging with a 1.5T MRI unit. We used this unit mainly for glioma (227) and pituitary (52) surgery.

## STANDARD PROCEDURES
### Open Craniotomies

Anesthesiology prepares the patient adjacent to the MR-suite. Then the patient is transported to the MR-OR suite. The head is fixed in a modified carbon-fiber, nonmagnetic, artifact-free Mayfield clamp (Promedics, Duesseldorf, Germany), which

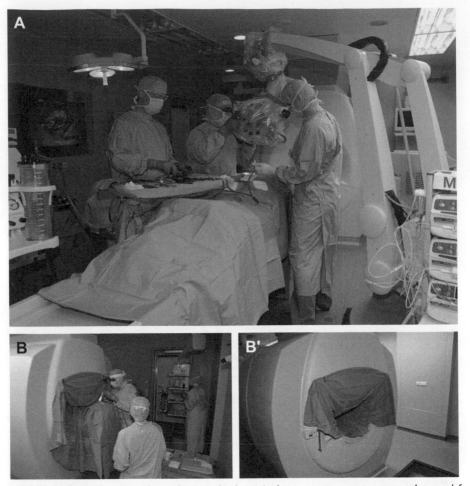

**Fig. 2.** Secondary surgical sites. Apart from the standard surgical area, two more areas can be used for specific indications. (*A*) The fringe field, which is at the border of the 5-G line (the red dot, between the assistant and the microscope base, symbolizes the 5-G line extension on the floor). Scrub and instruments are outside of the 5-G line. Right-hand corner: part of the anesthesiologist's equipment. Left side: the wall panel displays, showing the radiological data pertaining to the case or, as in this spinal tumor case, the microscope images. (*B*) Opposite to primary and fringe-field surgical area, at the back of the MRI. This area is within the 5-G line. We use a selected set of instruments, which are all MR-safe. Bipolar and ultrasonic aspirators can be used here, but not the microscope. This site is used for limited applications. However, scanning is even more comfortably integrated into the procedure since redraping is not necessary. The drapes are suspended from the MRI and the patient moved between surgical and imaging site as needed. Care must be taken that the drapes remain suspended. In this case, a 35-year-old patient underwent an open cortical biopsy. Various involved areas were interspersed with normal tissue. To ensure a representative sample, from the preoperatively identified MRI-target area, we performed the open biopsy "behind" the MRI. A lesion was unequivocally identified and removed.

is rigidly connected to the tabletop. We position the patient just outside of the MR tunnel. Although this is more cumbersome, it ensures that the patient fits inside the tunnel for scanning. One flexible surface coil is positioned below the patient's head, within the Mayfield clamp, while the other surface coil is placed on top. This coil is removed during surgery, and repositioned for scanning (on top of the draping). Earplugs are placed before the initial imaging. After positioning, we perform a T2-weighted scan, to rule out artifacts before

the patient is transferred to the surgical position. The dynamic reference frame (DRF) is fixed to the Mayfield clamp. It consists of two pieces, the base, firmly attached to the Mayfield and an upper portion. An interlocking mechanism ensures precise repositioning of the removable upper portion, holding the DRF. The navigation system is registered, the craniotomy planning finalized.

In the primary surgical area, ferromagnetic instruments can be used unhindered. After craniotomy, standard microneurosurgical techniques can be used for procedures such as tumor removal (see **Fig. 1**).

At the surgeon's discretion, repeat iMRI imaging is initiated. Every ferromagnetic item is removed and the surgical field is covered with additional sterile drapes. The table is returned to the MR-axis, connected, and the patient is transferred into the magnet (see **Fig. 1**). The surgeon analyses and reviews the data on the scanner console. The patient is then returned to the primary surgical area. The repeat iMRI scans are sent directly to the navigation system, and these new images are fused to the original data set, which was used for the initial referencing. With the DRF reattached in its original position, the images can be used for updated navigation without additional re-referencing (**Figs. 3** and **5B**). If residual tumor is identified, resection is continued, using the updated image data for continued neuronavigation. If no further resection is necessary, or deemed feasible, we conclude the surgery. A case with an anaplastic astrocytoma (World Health Organization III) is used to illustrate the quality of intraoperative images, the display on our navigation system, and decision making (**Figs. 4** and **5A, B**).

## Biopsies

Biopsies can be performed outside the 5-G line, using standard frame-based or frameless systems. Conventional frame-based stereotaxy allows the use of conventional tools with an MRI-compatible frame. Imaging is performed with the frame and localizer, and the images are transferred to a workstation to calculate the target coordinates. Subsequently the procedure is performed outside of the 5-G line, employing the standard instrumentation and technique. Confirmatory scans are acquired, with the frame in place, but the biopsy needle removed.

Frameless biopsy uses the ceiling-mounted integrated navigation system together with a specifically designed handpiece, which can be registered and tracked. Thus, the interactive mode can be used to guide the virtual advance of the needle. We use frameless techniques for the insertion of catheters for convection-enhanced delivery.

Both of these methods employ standard neurosurgical techniques and equipment. Furthermore, preoperative imaging, such as PET or single-photon emission computed tomography studies, can be integrated, yielding more date for target delineation. However, they lack the real-time guidance awarded by the in-bore technique.

Hall and Truwit have developed a method that integrates the MRI into the procedure. Termed "prospective stereotaxis," this method uses the magnet's online imaging capacity to target the lesion, monitor the needle's advance, and verify the correct position in real time.[17-21] The burr hole and dural opening are performed outside the 5-G line with conventional instrumentation. A burr hole-mounted, MRI-compatible[21] device is fixed, and the patient transferred to the scanner. The target is defined by structural and on-demand spectroscopic data. Subsequently the trajectory is planned.[18,20] The surgeon guides and advances the needle, standing at the cephalad end of the MRI, extending the arm into the bore. To provide

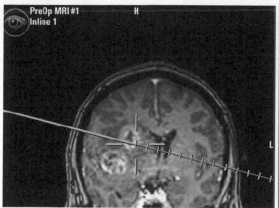 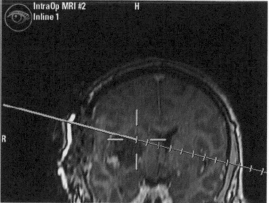

**Fig. 3.** Intraoperative update and demonstration of brain shift. Preoperative (*right*) and postoperative (*left*) coronal reformats of volumetric T1-WI. Patient with a multifocal glioblastoma. After resection, we re-referenced the acquired intraoperative data. The contrast-enhancing lesion was resected. The small contrast knot in the lower portion of the resection cavity was a bloody cottonoid. The navigation pointer is at the upper, medial resection margin (*left*) in the updated images whereas, judging by the preoperative images, the navigation's pointer tip would be at the bottom portion of the upper tumor portion.

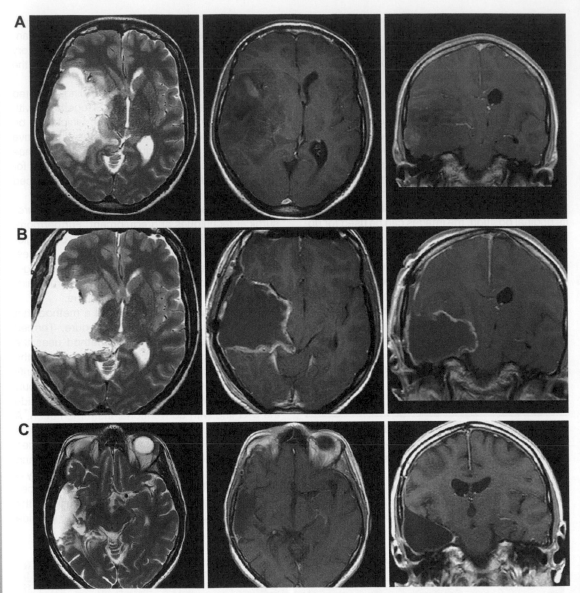

**Fig. 4.** Case study (continued in **Fig. 5**). Follow-up anaplastic astrocytoma (World Health Organization III) in a 42-year-old, right handed, female patient. (*A*) Preoperative scans: axial T2-WI showing the extension of the lesion, and the more diffuse pattern to the basal ganglia. The tumor extended even further along the temporal horn, toward the parietal lobe (as can be seen as residual lesion in C). T1-WI shows contrast enhancement in the lateral and temporopolar areas. Intraoperative T-WIs are displayed in **Fig. 5**A and intraoperative re-referenced images in **Fig. 5**B. (*B*) Postoperative images. Temporal lobe has been removed. Further nonenhancing tissue is extending adjacent to the basal ganglia and into the parietal lobe. The midline shift remains almost the same as before removal. Whereas DTI has been demonstrated in cases with large "rebound shift," in our case we see almost no deformation, representing some loss of elasticity. (*C*) Follow-up scans. The displaced midline and insular cortex have shifted back; diffuse tumor is visible in the parietal lobe. The brain stem has been decompressed; note the free upper tentorial notch.

real-time monitoring while advancing the needle, the imaging plane is chosen in plane to the trajectory. Image acquisitions of one to three images per second provide real-time control until the target is reached. Imaging confirming the correct position of the biopsy, and excluding complications ends

the procedure. The surgeon follows the real-time images on a ceiling-mounted monitor while handling the needle.

In the initial design, the biopsy needle was held and advanced manually. Further development provided remote control for this device, making it

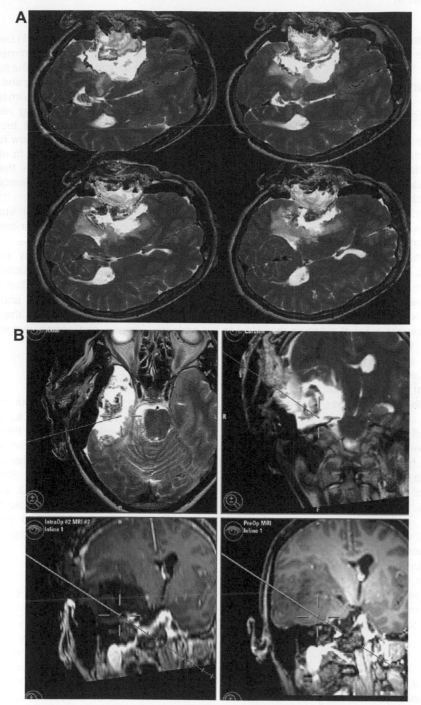

**Fig. 5.** (*A*) Intraoperative scan. Continued from **Fig. 4**. After a temporal lobe resection in the nondominant hemisphere, the resection was carried further, until most of the firmer, obviously tumorous areas were removed. The remainder was less clearly distinguishable. Intraoperative imaging confirmed suspected residual tumor. Risk analysis for removable tissue was based on this information. The herniating areas into the upper portion of the tentorial notch and the portion into the parietal lobe were targeted. The portions in the anterior aspect of the resection cavity and the medial portions extending into the basal ganglia were only partially addressed. (*B*) Screen shot from the updated navigation system. Upper two images show intraoperative T-WI mainly to depict the pyramidal tract. The left bottom image shows the intraoperative T-WI and the corresponding preoperative slice. The rigidity of the brain is impressive, remaining almost unchanged to the preoperative conformation. However, prejudiced by the major displacement preoperatively, manifest shift could have been expected. Here intraoperative imaging supplied valid information to continue resection and remove a significant portion of residual tumor.

more comfortable for the surgeon and more applicable to MRIs with less access to the patient.[20]

## BIOMECHANICAL PROPERTIES OF THE BRAIN

With the introduction of computer-assisted navigation systems a common surgical observation, intraoperative deformation of the brain, became an issue.[22] Intraoperative deformation, caused by various effects (eg, cerebrospinal fluid drainage, resection) invalidated presurgical data. While the ultimate resolution is intraoperative information renewal to update the neuronavigation,[13,14,23,24] various attempts were made to model and predict brain deformation patterns.[25–31]

Experimental and imaging data identified two distinct areas. The direction of deformation at the brain surface mostly follows gravity, sagging away from the surgeon. Subsurface deformation, however, is less predictable. Expansion due to swelling or, simply, relief of pressure may lead to deformation toward the resection cavity.[13,14] Again, in the example of a brain tumor, there are different patterns with primary gliomas and irradiated recurrent lesions, the latter showing less brain shift, potentially due to loss of elasticity after radiation.[14]

Whereas all these findings have been deduced from intraoperative imaging, prediction of tissue deformation has not yet been reliable. This is mainly due to the lack of information on elasticity coefficients of the brain. Being structured by white matter tracts, nuclei, and traversing vessels, it is conceivable why comprehensive models computing these factors and more physiologic data are imperfect.

Investigation of brain motion and elasticity are mandated to extract information on the biomechanical properties of the brain and to form a basis for the accurate implementation of computer programs to simulate brain shift.

## SUMMARY

Intraoperative high-field MRI is no longer a vision, but an established neurosurgical tool. Various methodologies have been implemented, applying mobile[6] and stationary scanners.[7,11] It is common to all described integrated MR-OR systems to have separated surgical and imaging space. Thus, the patient has to be transferred to the magnet or the magnet has to be brought the patient. Although this allows free access to the patient and higher image quality, this concept of separation makes serial scanning slightly cumbersome and navigational systems mandatory to use the data efficiently in surgery.[12] The question of how much time should be spent on intraoperative studies, and what immediate benefit they provide remains crucial for the surgical application of MRI. As long as imaging and surgery take place sequentially, intraoperative imaging remains a compromise balancing imaging versus surgical time. While microneurosurgical techniques are not hindered, the surgical workflow is interrupted. Although transfer is not lengthy in either MR-OR set-up, imaging, depending on the sequences chosen, may consume a considerable amount of time.

MR-ORs, which integrate MRI, state-of-the-art microneurosurgery and computer-assisted neuronavigation form a comprehensive unit for neurosurgical therapy. Whereas they provide many advances for visualization of structural and functional data, improved intraoperative neuronavigation with updated iMRI data, and information useful for the understanding of the "brain shift" problem, various challenges remain and some gain new importance.

## ACKNOWLEDGMENTS

Establishing an MRI-unit for our institution was a team effort. We are indebted to our OR-team. They have accepted the new "thing" and have made working in the MR-environment smoother, streamlining the workflow. We thank the Institute of Neuroradiology, in particular Stephan Ulmer, MD, and Olav Jansen, MD, PhD; our colleagues from the Department of Anesthesiology, in particular Dieter Hollander MD; and our colleagues from our Department of Neurosurgery.

## REFERENCES

1. Schenck JF, Jolesz FA, Roemer PB, et al. Superconducting open-configuration MR imaging system for image-guided therapy. Radiology 1995;195:805–14.
2. Tronnier VM, Wirtz CR, Knauth M, et al. Intraoperative diagnostic and interventional magnetic resonance imaging in neurosurgery. Neurosurgery 1997;40:891–900 [discussion: 900–2].
3. Steinmeier R, Fahlbusch R, Ganslandt O, et al. Intraoperative magnetic resonance imaging with the magnetom open scanner: concepts, neurosurgical indications, and procedures: a preliminary report. Neurosurgery 1998;43:739–47 [discussion: 747–8].
4. Black PM, Moriarty T, Alexander E III, et al. Development and implementation of intraoperative magnetic resonance imaging and its neurosurgical applications. Neurosurgery 1997;41:831–42 [discussion: 842–5].
5. Black PM, Alexander E III, Martin C, et al. Craniotomy for tumor treatment in an intraoperative

magnetic resonance imaging unit. Neurosurgery 1999;45:423–31 [discussion: 431–3].

6. Sutherland GR, Kaibara T, Louw D, et al. A mobile high-field magnetic resonance system for neurosurgery. J Neurosurg 1999;91:804–13.

7. Hall WA, Martin AJ, Liu H, et al. High-field strength interventional magnetic resonance imaging for pediatric neurosurgery. Pediatr Neurosurg 1998;29: 253–9.

8. Nimsky C, Ganslandt O, Fahlbusch R. Comparing 0.2 tesla with 1.5 tesla intraoperative magnetic resonance imaging analysis of setup, workflow, and efficiency. Acad Radiol 2005;12:1065–79.

9. Hall WA, Liu H, Maxwell RE, et al. Influence of 1.5-Tesla intraoperative MR imaging on surgical decision making. Acta Neurochir Suppl 2003;85:29–37.

10. Hall WA, Liu H, Martin AJ, et al. Safety, efficacy, and functionality of high-field strength interventional magnetic resonance imaging for neurosurgery. Neurosurgery 2000;46:632–41 [discussion: 641–2].

11. Nimsky C, Ganslandt O, von Keller B, et al. Preliminary experience in glioma surgery with intraoperative high-field MRI. Acta Neurochir Suppl 2003;88: 21–9.

12. Nimsky C, Ganslandt O, Buchfelder M, et al. Intraoperative visualization for resection of gliomas: the role of functional neuronavigation and intraoperative 1.5 T MRI. Neurol Res 2006;28:482–7.

13. Nimsky C, Ganslandt O, Cerny S, et al. Quantification of, visualization of, and compensation for brain shift using intraoperative magnetic resonance imaging. Neurosurgery 2000;47:1070–9 [discussion: 1079–80].

14. Nabavi A, Black PM, Gering DT, et al. Serial intraoperative magnetic resonance imaging of brain shift. Neurosurgery 2001;48:787–97 [discussion: 797–8].

15. Nimsky C, Ganslandt O, Von Keller B, et al. Intraoperative high-field-strength MR imaging: implementation and experience in 200 patients. Radiology 2004;233:67–78.

16. Kwan HC, Hazle JD, Jackson E, et al. In-vivo tissue characterization of brain by synthetic MR proton-relaxation and statistical chisquare parameter maps. Proceedings of the Eighth IEEE. Available at: http://ieeexplore.ieee.org/xpl/RecentCon.jsp?punumber=3237. Computer-Based Medical Systems; 1995. p. 338–45.

17. Hall WA, Martin A, Liu H, et al. Improving diagnostic yield in brain biopsy: coupling spectroscopic

18. Liu H, Hall WA, Martin AJ, et al. Biopsy needle tip artifact in MR-guided neurosurgery. J Magn Reson Imaging 2001;13:16–22.

19. Liu H, Hall WA, Truwit CL. Remotely-controlled approach for stereotactic neurobiopsy. Comput Aided Surg 2002;7:237–47.

20. Hall WA, Martin AJ, Liu H, et al. Brain biopsy using high-field strength interventional magnetic resonance imaging. Neurosurgery 1999;44:807–13 [discussion: 813–4].

21. Hall WA, Liu H, Truwit CL. Navigus trajectory guide. Neurosurgery 2000;46:502–4.

22. Roberts DW, Hartov A, Kennedy FE, et al. Intraoperative brain shift and deformation: a quantitative analysis of cortical displacement in 28 cases. Neurosurgery 1998;43:749–58 [discussion: 758–60].

23. Nimsky C, Ganslandt O, Hastreiter P, et al. Intraoperative compensation for brain shift. Surg Neurol 2001; 56:357–64 [discussion: 364–55].

24. Nabavi A, Gering DT, Kacher DF, et al. Surgical navigation in the open MRI. Acta Neurochir Suppl 2003; 85:121–5.

25. Hu J, Jin X, Lee JB, et al. Intraoperative brain shift prediction using a 3D inhomogeneous patient-specific finite element model. J Neurosurg 2007; 106:164–9.

26. Dumpuri P, Thompson RC, Dawant BM, et al. An atlas-based method to compensate for brain shift: preliminary results. Med Image Anal 2007;11:128–45.

27. Wittek A, Kikinis R, Warfield SK, et al. Brain shift computation using a fully nonlinear biomechanical model. Med Image Comput Comput Assist Interv Int Conf Med Image Comput Comput Assist Interv 2005;8:583–90.

28. Winkler D, Tittgemeyer M, Schwarz J, et al. The first evaluation of brain shift during functional neurosurgery by deformation field analysis. J Neurol Neurosurg Psychiatr 2005;76:1161–3.

29. Lunn KE, Paulsen KD, Lynch DR, et al. Assimilating intraoperative data with brain shift modeling using the adjoint equations. Med Image Anal 2005;9:281–93.

30. Clatz O, Delingette H, Talos IF, et al. Robust nonrigid registration to capture brain shift from intraoperative MRI. IEEE Trans Med Imaging 2005;24:1417–27.

31. Hastreiter P, Rezk-Salama C, Soza G, et al. Strategies for brain shift evaluation. Med Image Anal 2004;8:447–64.

# Three-Tesla High-Field Applications

Peter D. Kim, MD, PhD[a], Charles L. Truwit, MD[b,c],
Walter A. Hall, MD, MBA[a,*]

## KEYWORDS

- Magnetic resonance imaging
- Functional magnetic resonance imaging • Brain activation
- Brain biopsy • Brain neoplasms • Brain tumor

Modern neurosurgery depends greatly on neuroimaging. Although preoperative imaging provides sufficient information for the performance of many basic neurosurgical procedures, the advent of intraoperative CT guidance and frameless neuronavigation has allowed neurosurgeons to access smaller targets with less potential injury to adjacent normal brain. Intraoperative MRI (iMRI) has the advantages of near–real-time feedback coupled with high-resolution imaging and has been validated as a safe and cost-effective technique for brain tumor surgery and other neurosurgical procedures.[1] Additionally, iMRI does not have the major disadvantage of traditional neuronavigation techniques, namely, the loss of accuracy attributable to brain shift once the craniotomy is performed and the dura mater is opened.[2,3] During the resection of a brain tumor, after the bulk of the lesion is removed, the brain can shift toward the resection cavity and eloquent tissue may migrate into those areas previously occupied by tumor, potentially resulting in its resection if the surgeon were to rely solely on neuronavigation. Less frequent but also possible is the shift of tissue away from the surgical site attributable to the egress of cerebrospinal fluid or the contents of a cystic mass that allows residual tumor to move into an area thought to represent normal brain on preoperative navigation images.

The first iMRI scanner had a double-magnet configuration specifically designed for surgical use. The surgeon operated directly within the midfield 0.5-T magnet, and images could be obtained in an essentially continuous fashion.[4] Other low-field (<0.5 T) intraoperative scanners followed a similar design and were open MRI systems in which the magnet was adjacent to or descended below the surgical table.[5–8] The desire to improve image resolution and expand functional capabilities led to the development of high-field (1.5 T) iMRI suites.[9] These systems provided an increased signal-to-noise ratio but also created complex technical considerations, such as MRI compatibility, artifact generation, and spatial constraints. Compatibility is one of the greatest safety concerns, because traditional neurosurgical procedures are performed using a wide array of ferromagnetic instruments. Should a mishap occur in the presence of the high magnetic field, the potential for injury to the patient and staff and for damage to expensive imaging or surgical equipment is possible. Although this possibility is always a theoretic concern, the collective experience of those using iMRI systems has demonstrated that surgery in a high-field environment is safe. Additionally, neurosurgeons do not use low-field imaging for their preoperative evaluation, and many expect their iMRI, during which decisions must be made rapidly within the context of a changing anatomic background, to provide comparable high resolution.

The initial iMRI suite at the University of Minnesota consisted of a 1.5-T high-field scanner with which more than 1000 procedures were

[a] Department of Neurosurgery, State University of New York, Upstate Medical University, 750 East Adams Street, Syracuse, NY 13210, USA
[b] Department of Radiology, University of Minnesota Medical School, Minneapolis, MN, USA
[c] Department of Radiology, Hennepin County Medical Center, Minneapolis, MN, USA
* Corresponding author.
E-mail address: hallw@upstate.edu (W.A. Hall).

Neurosurg Clin N Am 20 (2009) 173–178
doi:10.1016/j.nec.2009.04.009

performed without any untoward safety events. Using the success of this system as a template, a 3-T ultra–high-field iMRI suite was designed and first used for the performance of brain biopsy in 2005.[10] Although the efficacy, cost-effectiveness, and ideal applications for 3-T iMRI are still unknown, the authors believe that 3-T iMRI is ultimately likely to become the standard of care for iMRI-guided neurosurgery because of the high resolution afforded and the advanced functional applications, such as brain activation studies, diffusion-weighted imaging, spectroscopy, and vascular imaging.

## THE SURGICAL SUITE

The suite must allow for an ergonomic operating field and a safe transition from the surgical environment to performing iMRI. Suites like the "double donut" arrangement, wherein the surgeon operates with the patient in the same position for imaging, offer a seamless transition but place constraints on the surgical environment. The use of an unmodified diagnostic scanner separated from a surgical area permits uncompromised operating space but at the cost of prolonging the imaging time and with the likelihood that fewer intraoperative scans can be obtained during the procedure. The original 1.5-T iMRI suite consisted of an MRI scanner separated from an operative area that was entirely outside the 5-G line. Most craniotomies were performed outside the 5-G line, allowing for the use of ferromagnetic instruments, although some minor procedures, such as brain biopsies, were performed at the back end of the scanner with MRI-compatible equipment. Although the time necessary to transport the patient between operating and scanning modalities can be minimized in the authors' experience and that of others, the need for multiple intraoperative scans can still lead to an increase in anesthesia time. Repeated transfer of the patient into the scanner also increases the potential for adverse events.

The increased strength of the 3-T magnet compared with that at 1.5-T necessitated that all the equipment in the iMRI suite be compatible with MRI. The Minnesota 3-T iMRI suite was therefore designed for surgery to be performed completely at the back end of the scanner with all MRI-compatible operative equipment. The need to perform the entire procedure in an MRI-compatible, or at least "MRI-acceptable," manner with the constraints of operating entirely within the confines of a diagnostic scanner represents the major challenge to transitioning from 1.5- to 3-T iMRI scanning. The authors believe that these

costs are worth the benefit and minimize the size of the operative suite, wherein the scanner and operative areas would otherwise be at opposite ends of the room. They have thus returned to a strategy in which surgery and scanning are accomplished without significant patient transport. Regardless of whether the operation takes place within the scanner or adjacent to the 5-G line within the same room, meticulous planning with the avoidance of ferromagnetic materials within the room is essential for the safe performance of procedures in the 3-T iMRI suite. MRI-compatible anesthesia equipment is available, and the authors have used the Aestiva 5/MRI ventilation and gas machine (Datex-Ohmeda, Helsinki, Finland) and 3155A and 3150 monitors (Invivo Intermagnetics, Orlando, Florida). The anesthesia column is installed adjacent to the back end of the scanner. The total size of the Minnesota 3-T suite is 1700 sq ft, whereas the operative area behind the scanner measures 167 sq ft. Positive pressure is maintained in the room to preserve the sterility of the surgical field. Finally, a surgical equipment room with a radiofrequency door and glass window houses the bipolar electrocautery, the foot pedal for the pneumatic drill, and the light source for the surgical headlight.

## THE SCANNER

Midfield intraoperative scanners were designed as dedicated surgical scanners. In addition to the original iMRI scanner, which featured a double-magnet design in which the surgeon was required to operate in the magnet, other dedicated iMRI systems included open low-field iMRI as previously described and a high-field (1.5 T) mobile iMRI system in which the magnet is suspended from the ceiling.[11]

Unlike these specially designed MRI systems, the authors adapted a routine diagnostic scanner for iMRI surgical use. The advantage of creating an operating suite for a fully functional diagnostic scanner is the reduction in costs, because the scanner may be used for traditional diagnostic radiology when not being used for surgery. Although the demand for iMRI continues to increase, the use of unaltered MRI equipment designed and produced for diagnostic purposes within adapted operating suites is likely to be the most affordable option for high-field applications for some time to come. The adaptation for surgery of the radiology suite containing a diagnostic scanner potentially allows any nonacademic or community institution with high-field MRI equipment to develop an iMRI surgical program.

The 3-T iMRI scanner measures 157 cm from front to back and 78.5 cm from the rear flared bore opening to the isocenter. The table may be extended 66 cm (33 cm as is, with an additional 33 cm from an extender designed for whole-body imaging) past the back opening of the scanner to allow for operating space (**Fig. 1**). One disadvantage of this 3-T setup is the inability to rotate the table around its short (left/right) or long (Trendelenburg/reverse Trendelenburg) axis. The patients must therefore be positioned in a way that can be achieved by bolstering the (generally supine) patient with gel rolls or bed sheets on a flat table.

An interactive scanning mode is enabled, which permits rapid single-slice acquisition in any plane. This imaging capability allows for near–real-time changes of scan planes and scanning parameters. The in-room liquid crystal display suspended from the ceiling can be rotated toward the surgeon and is located 100 cm from the back opening of the magnet.

## OPERATIVE PROCEDURES

Using the setup described previously, the authors have used the 3-T scanner for neurobiopsies (**Fig. 2**), lesion resection, and image-guided cyst aspiration. Pocketless color-coded scrubs are worn by all involved personnel to avoid the inadvertent introduction of ferromagnetic objects into the surgical suite. Patients are brought to the operating suite and, if needed, receive a preoperative scan while awake. When resecting enhancing

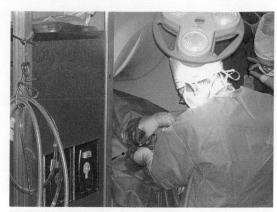

**Fig. 2.** Brain biopsy is performed at the back end of the 3-T MRI scanner. The MRI-compatible brain biopsy needle is clearly seen with the brake collar placed at the target depth. The anesthesia column is to the left, and the surgical light is overhead.

lesions, the administration of gadolinium is avoided during preoperative scanning to prevent diffusion of contrast into the brain parenchyma around the lesion, which would make interpretation of the intraoperative scans difficult. Patients receive general endotracheal anesthesia using MRI-compatible equipment. The head is secured on a rubber donut with tape, because a rigid three-point fixation device that has been designed for 3-T iMRI use is not available. The incision is made using a plastic-handled scalpel (Sandel safety scalpel; Sandel Medical, Chatsworth, California) whose metal blade, although ferromagnetic, has a magnetic pull less than gravity as long as it is kept at least 38 cm away from the magnet. Even within a 38-cm radius, the magnetic pull is easily controlled by the surgeon. Suture needles are also carefully controlled while in the surgical field to prevent projection attributable to magnetic influence. For biopsy, the technique of prospective stereotaxy is used.[12] After placement of the burr hole, a trajectory guide (Medtronic, St. Paul, Minnesota) is anchored in place with self-tapping screws. Once the target has been identified, two additional points are defined: the pivot point at the tip of the alignment stem and the third point that represents the desired location for the cross section of the alignment stem. When all three points are colinear, the biopsy needle encounters the target. Once these points are aligned, scanning along the axis of the alignment stem is performed to confirm that the needle can be guided toward the target (**Fig. 3**). Once this is confirmed, the locking nut of the trajectory guide is tightened, the alignment stem is removed, and the needle is slowly advanced while images are obtained periodically. When the needle

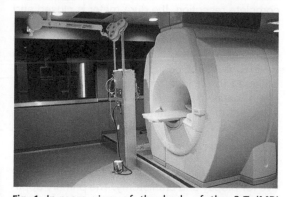

**Fig. 1.** In-room view of the back of the 3-T iMRI scanner that measures 157 cm from front to back and 78.5 cm from the rear flared bore opening to the isocenter. The table is extended 33 cm past the back opening of the scanner to allow for operating space in the recessed surgical pit. Note the anesthesia column located to the left of the scanner and the overhead surgical light. The liquid crystal display monitor is reflected in the window of a conference room that is used for viewing surgical procedures.

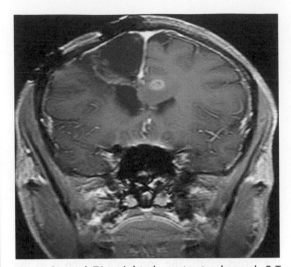

**Fig. 3.** Coronal T1-weighted, contrast-enhanced, 3-T MRI scan shows an enhancing lesion located in the left frontal lobe thought to be tumor spread across the corpus callosum. The patient previously had an oligodendroglioma resected in the right frontal lobe. The resection cavity and craniotomy site are seen on the right.

encounters the target, it is locked in place, orthogonal oblique scans (**Fig. 4**) are acquired in two planes for confirmation, and the patient is advanced out of the scanner to obtain the biopsy

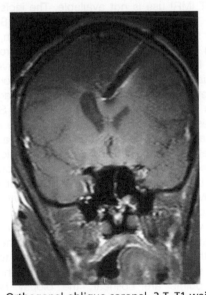

**Fig. 4.** Orthogonal oblique coronal, 3-T, T1-weighted, contrast-enhanced scan oriented along the entire length of the MRI-compatible titanium biopsy needle, which has encountered the target lesion. The indentation near the end of the biopsy needle represents the proximal end of the side-cutting port. Note the degree of artifact associated with the biopsy needle in this spatial orientation. The biopsy revealed an anaplastic oligodendroglioma.

tissue. While frozen section analysis is ongoing, the needle is removed, leaving the brake collar in place in case there is a need for additional tissue sampling. Postbiopsy scanning is also performed to exclude the presence of radiographically or clinically significant hemorrhage. The need to exclude hyperacute blood, which can be difficult to visualize on MRI, has led the authors to obtain half-Fourier acquisition single-shot turbo spin-echo (HASTE), gradient echo T2*, and turbo fluid-attenuated inversion recovery (FLAIR) sequences when scanning during surgery to exclude hemorrhage.

The procedure for open craniotomy is similar in most aspects to that of biopsy. The anesthetized patient is secured with adhesive tape on the table with the head on a foam-rubber donut. One radiofrequency coil is placed directly under the head, and a second is placed on the head away from the operative site. The draping and incision are the same as with the biopsy. The craniotomy is performed using an MRI-compatible pneumatic drill. When operative imaging is thought to be indicated, the bipolar electrocautery and suction equipment are placed on the back table and the patient is moved to bring the surgical field to the isocenter of the scanner. The operative field is continuously visualized during this short transfer to ensure that there is no breach in sterility. Intravenous contrast is administered for intraoperative scans before the acquisition of T1 imaging. The presence of any residual enhancement could be an indication for further resection, with repeat intraoperative scanning performed when the surgeon believes that the residual enhancing tissue has been resected. Once scanning confirms complete resection, the dura mater is closed and the bone flap is replaced using an MRI-compatible plating system (Osteomed, Dallas, Texas). The craniotomy is closed, and one final scan with HASTE, gradient echo, and turbo-FLAIR MRI is obtained to exclude the presence of intracranial hemorrhage. The patient is extubated in the MRI suite and then brought to the recovery room.

## FUTURE DIRECTIONS

iMRI has been demonstrated to be safe and effective for biopsy and craniotomy. The primary application of iMRI guidance has been for intracerebral tumor resection, and there is justification in the literature in combination with experiential evidence that iMRI guidance increases the likelihood of achieving gross total tumor resection.[13] With an increasing body of literature accumulating in support of the survival benefit derived from gross total resection for low- and high-grade gliomas,[14–17] iMRI should continue to play an increasing role in the treatment of these tumors. The next generation of high-field iMRI studies may be functional, such as for the acquisition of brain activation studies to guide the resection of tumors near eloquent cortex (**Fig. 5**) and in guiding the placement of neurostimulators. Three-Tesla imaging offers superior functional MRI (fMRI) data compared with those obtained at 1.5 T and permits the demonstration of cortical activation on multiple slices. The authors' previous paradigm for fMRI-guided neurosurgery has been to acquire brain activation studies before surgery using a dedicated 1.5- or 3-T diagnostic scanner, followed by performing the craniotomy using 1.5-T iMRI guidance. Brain activation imaging or blood oxygen-level dependent fMRI was used to determine the location of motor function and speech function. Tasks for motor function included finger and toe tapping, whereas for language, silent speech was performed to avoid motion artifact from actual speaking. Using this paradigm, tumors located near eloquent cortex were resected without permanent neurologic deficits in any patient. The authors' initial experience was with fMRI acquisition at 1.5 T, followed by iMRI guidance also at 1.5 T. They have previously reported on this series of patients who had low-grade

gliomas.[18] This report was followed by a report on a second series of patients who underwent 3-T fMRI data acquisition before resection or biopsy in the 1.5-T iMRI suite.[19] In both series, no patient experienced a permanent neurologic injury, despite the fact that all had tumors located adjacent to eloquent cortex.

Using a 3-T iMRI scanner would obviate the need for acquiring functional data in a separate session. The ability to obtain brain activation studies in the immediate preoperative period would offer the benefit of streamlined processing and provide the most current scans possible. Once again, the consistency of matching the resolution of the intraoperative scans with the functional and preoperative imaging has an obvious appeal.

Placement of deep brain stimulators (DBSs) would be another ideal application for high-field iMRI guidance. Because extremely accurate electrode placement within small brain nuclei is necessary to optimize outcome in nearly all neurostimulation procedures, the resolution provided by 3-T high-field intraoperative scanning should be useful. Whether iMRI guidance could replace microelectrode recording or would typically be used as an adjuvant measure for electrode placement is difficult to predict. If microelectrode mapping could be circumvented by using iMRI, this would spare the patient performance of surgery while awake, in addition to multiple passes of the microelectrode through the brain with the concomitant risk for hemorrhage and significantly increased length of the operative time required. The patient could also undergo DBS placement without a drug holiday, which is required when placing a DBS with microelectrode guidance. Initial data suggest that iMRI may be sufficient alone for placement of a DBS. A prospective study of 20 patients in which prospective stereotaxy was used to target the subthalamic nucleus for patients who had Parkinson disease found a high success rate, with an average distance of less than 1 mm between predicted and postoperative MRI coordinates.[20] Similarly, iMRI with prospective stereotaxy was used to guide DBS placement in 42 patients who had Parkinson disease or dystonia.[21] Once again, the difference between the planned and actual trajectories was small (1.2 mm), and electrode placement was accomplished with one pass 90% of the time. The advantage of providing prospective guidance in addition to confirmation is thus a major benefit of using iMRI for DBS placement. Another advantage of iMRI guidance is the ability to exclude the presence of hemorrhage at the time of electrode placement. Although most reported series of iMRI-guided neurostimulator

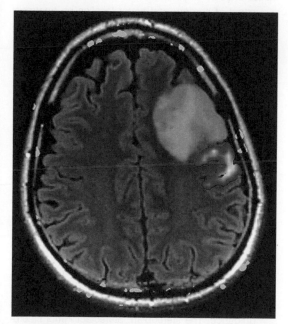

**Fig. 5.** Axial turbo-FLAIR 3-T MRI scan shows the area of brain activation associated with finger tapping of the right hand. The location of eloquent function is immediately posterior to an area of increased signal that was found to be an oligodendroglioma on histopathologic examination. After what was thought to be a complete radiographic resection, the patient had no postoperative speech or motor deficits.

placement are at 1.5 T, 3-T high-field iMRI would offer the advantage of higher resolution. Challenges would be to overcome the artifact that is generated by the microelectrodes sufficiently to allow for precise determination of their placement location. At present, the manufacturer's guidelines state that only MRI at 1.5 T should be performed on patients with these systems. High-field iMRI for DBS placement is likely to be limited to this magnet strength for some time.

## SUMMARY

The authors believe that 3-T iMRI is eventually likely to become the standard of care for a wide range of neurosurgical procedures. Although 3-T high-field image acquisition does pose challenges, the advantages of this field strength, such as superior visualization of soft tissue and clear delineation of any residual enhancing tissue, are clearly optimized using this equipment. Additionally, the use of 3-T high-field scanning offers functional options, such as brain activation studies and complex vascular imaging, that are unavailable with low- and midfield iMRI systems. The authors believe that the cost and effort necessary to acquire and establish a 3-T high-field iMRI program represent the natural progression for image-guided neurosurgery.

## REFERENCES

1. Kucharczyk J, Hall WA, Broaddus WC, et al. Cost-efficacy of MR-guided neurointerventions. Neuroimaging Clin N Am 2001;11(4):767–72.
2. Trantakis C, Tittgemeyer M, Schneider JP, et al. Investigation of time-dependency of intracranial brain shift and its relation to the extent of tumor removal using intra-operative MRI. Neurol Res 2003;25(1):9–12.
3. Reinges MH, Nguyen HH, Krings T, et al. Course of brain shift during microsurgical resection of supratentorial cerebral lesions: limits of conventional neuronavigation. Acta Neurochir (Wien) 2004;146(4):369–77.
4. Schwartz RB, Hsu L, Wong TZ, et al. Intraoperative MR imaging guidance for intracranial neurosurgery: experience with the first 200 cases. Radiology 1999; 211(2):477–88.
5. Tronnier VM, Wirtz CR, Knauth M, et al. Intraoperative diagnostic and interventional magnetic resonance imaging in neurosurgery. Neurosurgery 1997;40(5):891–900.
6. Rubino GJ, Farahani K, McGill D, et al. Magnetic resonance imaging-guided neurosurgery in the magnetic fringe fields: the next step in neuronavigation. Neurosurgery 2000;46(3):643–53.
7. Schulder M, Catrambone J, Carmel PW. Intraoperative magnetic resonance imaging at 0.12 T: is it enough? Neurosurg Clin N Am 2005;16(1):143–54.
8. Muragaki Y, Iseki H, Maruyama T, et al. Usefulness of intraoperative magnetic resonance imaging for glioma surgery. Acta Neurochir Suppl 2006;98: 67–75.
9. Hall WA, Liu H, Maxwell RE, et al. Influence of 1.5-Tesla intraoperative MR imaging on surgical decision making. Acta Neurochir Suppl 2003;85:29–37.
10. Truwit CL, Hall WA. Intraoperative magnetic resonance imaging-guided neurosurgery at 3-T. Neurosurgery 2006;58(4 Suppl 2):338–46.
11. Sutherland GR, Kaibara T, Louw D, et al. A mobile high-field magnetic resonance system for neurosurgery. J Neurosurg 1999;91(5):804–13.
12. Hall WA, Truwit CL. 1.5 T: spectroscopy-supported brain biopsy. Neurosurg Clin N Am 2005;16(1): 165–72.
13. Knauth M, Wirtz CR, Tronnier VM, et al. Intraoperative MR imaging increases the extent of tumor resection in patients with high-grade gliomas. AJNR Am J Neuroradiol 1999;20(9):1642–6.
14. Berger MS, Deliganis AV, Dobbins J, et al. The effect of extent of resection on recurrence in patients with low grade cerebral hemisphere gliomas. Cancer 1994;74(6):1784–91.
15. Jeremic B, Grujicic D, Antunovic V, et al. Influence of extent of surgery and tumor location on treatment outcome of patients with glioblastoma multiforme treated with combined modality approach. J Neuro-oncol 1994;21(2):177–85.
16. Buckner JC. Factors influencing survival in high-grade gliomas. Semin Oncol 2003;30(6 Suppl 19): 10–4.
17. Vidiri A, Carapella CM, Pace A, et al. Early postoperative MRI: correlation with progression-free survival and overall survival time in malignant gliomas. J Exp Clin Cancer Res 2006;25(2): 177–82.
18. Hall WA, Liu H, Truwit CL. Functional magnetic resonance imaging-guided resection of low-grade gliomas. Surg Neurol 2005;64(1):20–7.
19. Hall WA, Truwit CL. 3-Tesla functional magnetic resonance imaging-guided tumor resection. Int J CARS 2007;1:223–30.
20. Derrey S, Maltête D, Chastan N, et al. Deep brain stimulation of the subthalamic nucleus in Parkinson's Disease: usefulness of intraoperative radiological guidance. The stereoplan. Stereotact Funct Neurosurg 2008;86(6):351–8.
21. Martin AJ, Hall WA, Roark C, et al. Minimally invasive precision brain access using prospective stereotaxy and a trajectory guide. J Magn Reson Imaging 2008; 27:737–43.

# Software Requirements for Interventional MR in Restorative and Functional Neurosurgery

Alastair J. Martin, PhD[a],*, Philip A. Starr, MD, PhD[b],
Paul S. Larson, MD[b]

**KEYWORDS**

- Imaging • Magnetic resonance
- Software • Neuronavigation • Functional neurosurgery

MRI plays a key diagnostic role in restorative and functional neurosurgery. It is the imaging modality of choice for visualizing brain structures and can provide crucial feedback on therapeutic responses based on anatomic, functional, or spectroscopic evaluations. The evolution of MR methods into the operative setting, however, creates many new challenges and opportunities. The MR system and operator must adapt to the temporal and sterility demands of the operative setting. Furthermore, the surgery staff must adapt to the MR environment, including the safety implications and periods of inactivity during MRI acquisitions. It is therefore crucial that pre- and intraoperative imaging information be efficiently acquired and seamlessly presented to the surgical team. One of the most important elements to integrating MRI to the operative setting is, therefore, the software that controls the MR acquisition, processes the image data, and subsequently presents the new information to the surgical team.

This article discusses the software requirements for applying interventional MRI (iMRI) techniques to restorative and functional neurosurgery. The authors initially present an example of the use of real-time iMRI techniques to accurately target deep brain structures. This application serves to highlight the need for optimized software and identifies the limitations of existing iMRI consoles for this application. The authors subsequently explore the properties of present neuronavigation platforms and evolving iMRI interfaces to define a software environment that is appropriate for performing restorative and functional neurosurgery under iMRI guidance.

## MR IN RESTORATIVE AND FUNCTIONAL NEUROSURGERY

MR techniques have been introduced into neurosurgical settings since the early 1990s.[1] The vast majority of these iMRI studies, however, have been aimed at open surgical procedures, such as tumor resections. The role of the MR system in these types of procedures is much like a still camera, with images capturing surgical progress at distinct stages. Imaging and surgery are thus largely independent, and MR data can be acquired in conventional fashions and forwarded to existing neuronavigation platforms for guidance between imaging updates. This approach inherently requires registration of the MR images with the surgical field, which takes time and has limited accuracy. It has the advantage of the operative

a Department of Radiology and Biomedical Imaging, University of California San Francisco, Box 0628, Room L-310, 505 Parnassus Avenue, San Francisco, CA 94143, USA
b Department of Neurological Surgery, University of California San Francisco, Room 779M, 505 Parnassus Avenue, San Francisco, CA 94143, USA
* Corresponding author.
E-mail address: alastair.martin@radiology.ucsf.edu (A.J. Martin).

Neurosurg Clin N Am 20 (2009) 179–186
doi:10.1016/j.nec.2009.04.003
1042-3680/09/$ – see front matter © 2009 Elsevier Inc. All rights reserved.

and imaging periods being largely distinct, resulting in the adoption of iMRI systems that can be brought to the surgical field only when they are needed and withdrawn otherwise.[2,3] This approach also has limitations, in that the MR images cannot reflect or visualize dynamic changes that occur during surgery.

Minimally invasive surgical techniques have significant benefits but often suffer from a limited ability to visualize the operative field. This compromised direct visual inspection frequently dictates that alternate surgical guidance be used. Stereotaxy is routinely used in these circumstances and involves the creation of a reliable frame of reference against which imaging data and surgical manipulations can be registered. This process can either be achieved with a frame that is secured to a patient's skull (framed stereotaxy) or by the identification of landmarks that are readily recognized on both images and the patient (frameless stereotaxy). The methodology then requires a means of directing a surgical instrument toward the target identified in the frame of reference, which can either be performed with a physical arc system that is attached to a rigid stereotactic frame or with a navigation platform that can visualize the geometric properties of surgical devices with respect to the image data. The latter usually involves optical tracking of the patient and surgical instruments. Conventional stereotaxy is based on preoperative images that cannot account for ongoing brain shift during a procedure and is technically complex and subject to user error, so it does not by itself always provide the required accuracy for many applications in functional neurosurgery. Alternate methodologies, such as microelectrode recording (MER) in the case of lesioning procedures or deep brain stimulation (DBS), are used to infer position intraoperatively.[4,5] MER, for instance, achieves spatial sensitivity based on the characteristic firing patterns of neurons in different regions of the brain. The information provided by these intraoperative methodologies may be complimentary to image data, but may also provide contradictory or confounding results. They further frequently require invasive approaches, such as the introduction of an electrode into the brain in the case of MER. There is substantial interest in intraoperative MR imaging that could provide guidance and feedback for minimally invasive functional neurosurgery procedures.

### Implantation of Deep Brain Stimulators

Preliminary studies using iMRI methods to guide functional neurosurgery have been performed. These include MR-guided ablative therapies[6,7]

and implantation of DBS electrodes.[8,9] The methodologies that have been developed for iMRI-guided interventions are potentially applicable to a wide range of other functional and restorative therapies that require precision access to deep brain structures. Localized delivery of drug, gene, or cell therapies may require or benefit from highly localized delivery and visualization of agent distribution patterns. There is great interest in further developing techniques and tools for iMRI guidance of an assortment of minimally invasive approaches.

The specific methodology that was developed for DBS implantation is an excellent example of the novel surgical approaches that are applied in iMRI. This technique is described elsewhere in this issue in detail, but in brief it involves a custom burr hole–mounted trajectory guide that contains components that are both MR compatible and MR visible. A technique that is referred to as prospective stereotaxy[10,11] is then used to align the trajectory guide toward the selected target (**Fig. 1**).

This general approach has been used to deliver more than 50 electrodes into the subthalamic nucleus of Parkinsonian patients with good technical outcomes.[12] The procedure is actually performed within the magnet bore (**Fig. 2**) and it takes advantage of the imaging volume being inherently fused to the patient's anatomy. Ideally a marking grid would be placed on the patient and a surface-rendered view of the skin/grid surface obtained to mark the desired site for burr hole creation. Following the trajectory guide mounting, the MR scanner must prescribe imaging planes that precisely contain the intended trajectory in multiple, usually orthogonal, views. This function is typically performed graphically, although it is also possible to manually input specific scan plane coordinates. The former is subject to small inaccuracies, whereas the latter is tedious and subject to input errors. Scan planes that are automatically generated based on the coordinate system of the target (ie, anterior commissure-posterior commissure (AC-PC) space) or the specified trajectory would be highly desirable. The MR scanner must further be capable of determining the orientation of the trajectory guide and project the path through the brain that would be produced. The latter requires segmentation of the external alignment indicator and a fit of its linear orientation, neither of which is typically available on MR consoles. Finally, the software must be able to monitor the passage of the device through the brain and determine its position with respect to the intended target. Existing MR software is largely adequate for this purpose, although an additional evaluation of

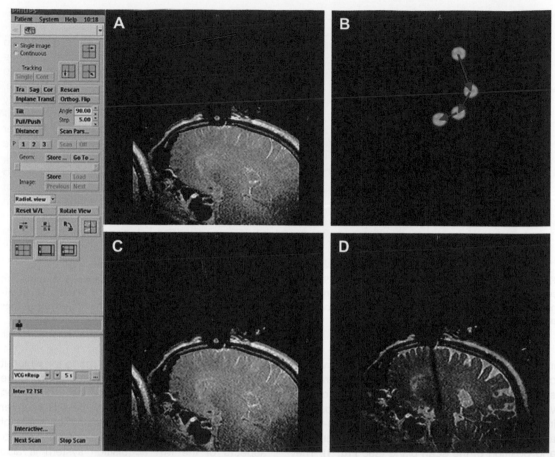

**Fig. 1.** The imaging methodology that is used for DBS implantation is summarized. A scan plane is initially defined that contains the desired trajectory (*A*). The trajectory guide is then aligned by imaging in a scan plane that is centered on the desired trajectory and positioned above the head, where only the alignment indicator is visible (scan plane is indicated with the red line in *A*). Fluoroscopic MR imaging is then used to manipulate the trajectory guide until it is collinear with the desired trajectory (*B*). Once suitably aligned, the trajectory is confirmed (*C*), and a rigid ceramic mandrel is inserted to the target (*D*). These stages are all demonstrated within a real-time interactive interface, which permits visualization of these dynamic processes and is commercially available on most MR systems.

precise device position and orientation throughout this process is desirable.

## EXISTING SOFTWARE INTERFACES

There are numerous software interfaces that are used for acquiring MR images, postprocessing acquired images, fusing data from multiple sources, and image display during surgery. The specific software requirements depend strongly on the primary activities that are anticipated and therefore can vary widely between consoles. Moche and colleagues[13] provide a detailed overview of navigation concepts that are applied to iMRI, but we focus here on software that is specifically relevant to functional and restorative neurosurgery.

## MR Consoles

MR data are largely viewed as stacks of two-dimensional images and are commonly shipped to centralized picture archive and communication systems for image interpretation, review, sharing, and storage. As such, the MR software environment is primarily image prescription and acquisition oriented, with an assortment of basic postprocessing functions incorporated. This functionality is well suited to seeding stereotactic approaches, but is not optimal for surgical settings, where acquisition, processing, and display must occur rapidly. Real-time MR imaging capabilities are becoming available, either directly on the MR console or as part of specialized control workstations that operate in parallel with the MR

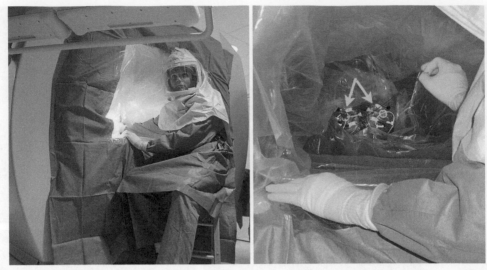

**Fig. 2.** A surgeon performing a bilateral DBS implantation with intraoperative MR guidance is shown. The surgeon operates at the back of an MR scanner (*left*) and reaches into the magnet bore to manipulate skull-mounted trajectory guides (*arrows in right panel*). Real-time scanning is used to align the trajectory guides and monitor device insertion.

interface. Yutzy and Duerk[14] recently reviewed commercial offerings of real time, or interactive, software environments offered by major MR vendors. These interfaces permit fluoroscopic imaging in multiple scan planes and on-the-fly adjustment to image contrast and the orientation and position of the scan plane (see **Fig. 1**). They thus permit real-time control over scan prescription and immediately display planar images as they are acquired. They are largely limited to single-slice views, however, and little image manipulation or processing is possible.

A software interface capable of live three-dimensional renderings has been developed and customized for the interventional MR environment.[15] This software was developed on a stand-alone workstation and was specifically aimed at cardiovascular iMRI procedures. The workstation was connected by Ethernet directly to the image reconstruction computer of the MR system to minimize latency between image acquisition and display on this independent workstation. The MR system was further programmed to accept a host of scan prescription commands from the independent workstation, creating a customized interventional platform that could control basic aspects of image acquisition and provide optimal display. The advantage of this type of approach is that the software on the external workstation can be adapted to the specific needs of an interventional procedure without having to affect the operational software and database architecture of a conventional MR system. The MR system

can continue to operate in the mode for which it has been optimized, which is focused on image acquisition, while the stand-alone workstation processes the data emitted by the MR scanner to provide the desired visualization. The ability of this external workstation to directly control aspects of the MR acquisition system is also appealing, although this presently requires adaptation of the MR software.

### Neuronavigation Systems

Navigation systems (StealthStation, Medtronic Inc., Minneapolis, Minnesota; VectorVision Brain-LAB AG, Heimstetten, Germany) offer a wealth of visualization capabilities based largely on registered MR or CT volumes, but are usually off-line from the acquisition system (**Fig. 3**).

These systems are unique in that they combine hardware (fiducial markers, optical systems, specialized instruments) and a software environment to provide a fully integrated and stand-alone stereotactic system. The software therefore serves two functions: (1) to perform registration of the patient anatomy with the preoperative imaging, and (2) to allow real-time navigation during the procedure. The strength of the software in neuronavigation systems is its ability to display reconstructed images in multiple planes simultaneously and rapidly in ways that are helpful and intuitive to the surgeon. The user can view images in anatomic planes or planes relative to various instruments or probes in real time.

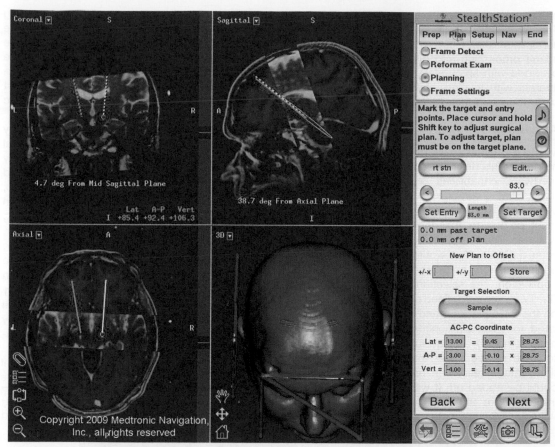

**Fig. 3.** A screen grab captured from a StealthStation (Medtronic) during planning of the insertion of DBS electrodes. The patient is secured in a stereotactic frame and preoperative MR data are registered to this coordinate system. The surgeon can visualize the MR images in several reformatted planes to plan the surgical approach. (*Courtesy of* Medtronic Navigation, Louisville, CO; with permission. Copyright © 2009, Medtronic Navigation Inc. All rights reserved.)

Surgical plans can also be created by the user to define a target, entry point, and trajectory before the procedure, and these plans can be used to monitor the apparent accuracy and progress of the surgery. Such feedback has become the standard of care in many modern-day neurosurgical suites.

There are, however, limitations to using preoperative data for navigation purposes. The performance of any interventional procedure inherently requires interaction with the patient and this can result in geometric changes to the patient's anatomy that are not reflected in the preoperative data. Cerebrospinal fluid loss and the introduction of air into the cranial space following burr hole preparation and dura penetration has been shown to result in brain distortion.[16] Attempts to predict and correct for brain deformation with readily available intraoperative imaging (ultrasound) have been undertaken with some efficacy.[17] Coregistration of preoperative data with the patient in the operating room and any readily available

intraoperative imaging (ie, ultrasound) has fundamentally limited accuracy, however.[18] These registration errors can be highly relevant in functional neurosurgical procedures and appropriate steps must be taken to avoid their introduction or overcome their impact. It would thus be desirable to integrate the visualization capabilities of these neuronavigation platforms with optimal intraoperative imaging. Indeed, some IMR manufacturers now have integrated surgical navigation systems into their platforms to allow navigation using serially updated images from the MR scanner.

## SOFTWARE ENVIRONMENT OF THE FUTURE

An ideal software environment for restorative and functional neurosurgery would require a fusion of the MR acquisition system with the intuitive visualization capabilities of neuronavigation platforms. It would further need to synthesize existing stand-alone technologies into a real-time interface that permits immediate and intuitive feedback based on completed or even ongoing MR acquisitions. The software would ideally control relevant aspects of image acquisition and all aspects of image processing and display. Users should be provided with an intuitive interface that they can interact with to plan, execute, and evaluate the performance of their surgical procedure.

## Acquisition

MR is a phenomenally rich and diverse imaging modality. This diversity, coupled with specific MR hardware capabilities and limitations, creates substantial complexity in defining pulse sequences. Many details of MR pulse sequences must be left to the host computer of the MR scanner. There are, however, basic aspects of scan definition that would greatly benefit if they originated from software dedicated to the iMRI application. The selection of basic MR contrasts ($T_1$, $T_2$, $T_2^*$) or predefined protocols could originate on the iMRI platform and subsequently be translated to pulse sequences executed by the MR host computer. It may further be advantageous to have simple slider interfaces whereby scan time, image resolution and signal-to-noise ratio could be traded off. It will, however, be critically important for the iMRI software to control the volume of coverage and the offsets and

angulations of image acquisitions. The imaging volume and its orientation will all be driven by the needs of the surgical procedure and may require precise positioning for the surgical goals to be achieved. It is therefore logical that the iMRI workstation operate as the master and the MR host computer the slave for defining the geometric properties of image acquisitions.

The interface with the data stream emitted by the MR acquisition system will also be a crucial factor for the iMRI software to handle. In many instances, MR acquisitions can be completed and DICOM data, with full header information, sent from the MR system to the iMRI software. In situations in which fluoroscopic imaging is being used to monitor dynamic processes, however, this level of data access will be insufficient. Rather, the iMRI software will require access to the image data as they are emitted by the reconstruction computer of the MR system. These data typically have minimal header information and the iMRI software must be able to anticipate and properly interpret the data that are emitted by the reconstruction computer.

## Processing

In many instances acquired data must be processed to provide the most meaningful and

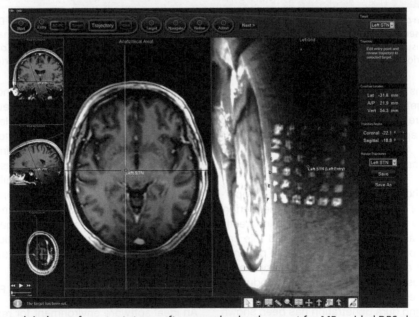

**Fig. 4.** A screen grab is shown from prototype software under development for MR-guided DBS electrode implantation. The software allows the user to select a target (*middle panel*) and then visualize potential trajectories to the target (*left panel*) in a manner analogous to conventional navigation platforms. It permits surface-rendered and cut-away views (*right panel*) that are conveyed to the surgeon in an intuitive format consistent with the surgeon's perspective of the patient. The software further allows blending of intraoperatively acquired single-slice or slab acquisitions on volumetric data and has dedicated tools for aligning a trajectory guide and evaluating device insertion into the brain. (*Courtesy of* Surgi-Vision, Inc.; with permission.)

informative perspectives to the surgeon. There frequently must be the ability to interact with volumetric data in real time, with seamless reformatting, surface rendering (**Fig. 4**), or volumetric rendering of the MR data as required. The acquisition of updated MR data, be they single-slice, multislice, or volumetric, must then be registered or fused with previously acquired data to provide a comprehensive overview of the current status of the patient and interventional devices. There may additionally be benefit to the incorporation of anatomic atlases or automatic detection of anatomic landmarks, fiducials, or surgical devices. These must all occur rapidly and the surgeon must have the opportunity to interact with the acquired data in the manner that they see fit. These features are already available on many neuronavigation systems, but the iMRI software will also be required to handle dynamic image updates and continuously integrate these data into the images being presented to the surgeon. This may require that the operator lock a specific view for monitoring the dynamically acquired data, but the ability to augment visualization of the dynamic data with previously acquired or processed data should be retained.

## Display

Presentation of acquired and processed MR data is a crucial responsibility of any iMRI software package. Display will typically occur on a monitor within the magnet room of the MR system, although other circumstances could also be envisioned. This display station will typically have minimal controls because of sterility requirements and the surgeon should be able to adequately control the workstation with this interface. Acquired MR data should typically be displayed with the same perspective that the surgeon has of the patient, although full flexibility in viewing must be available. The display should be able to present not only imaging data but also other crucial aspects of the procedure, such as patient physiologic status.

The concept of augmented reality,[19] which has already been applied to the iMRI environment,[20] may also be desirable for optimally fusing imaging data with actual patient anatomy. Augmented reality systems aim to simultaneously visualize the patient and image data and use stereoscopic glasses onto which the image data are projected. These display interfaces, although still in early development stages, hold great potential for truly fusing the surgeon's physical perspective of the patient with the host of imaging data that can be obtained.

## SUMMARY

iMRI holds great promise for optimally guiding and monitoring restorative and functional neurosurgical procedures. This technology has already been used to guide ablative therapies and insert DBS electrodes, and many future applications are envisioned. An optimized software interface is crucial for efficiently integrating the imaging data acquired during these procedures. MR systems are largely dedicated to image prescription and acquisition, whereas neuronavigation systems typically operate with previously acquired static data. An optimal software interface for iMRI requires fusion of many of the capabilities offered by these individual devices, and further requires the development of tools to handle the integration and presentation of dynamically updated data.

## REFERENCES

1. Black PM, Moriarty T, Alexander E 3rd, et al. Development and implementation of intraoperative magnetic resonance imaging and its neurosurgical applications. Neurosurgery 1997;41(4):831–42 [discussion: 842–35].
2. Kanner AA, Vogelbaum MA, Mayberg MR, et al. Intracranial navigation by using low-field intraoperative magnetic resonance imaging: preliminary experience. J Neurosurg 2002;97(5):1115–24.
3. Sutherland GR, Kaibara T, Louw DF. Intraoperative MR at 1.5 Tesla—experience and future directions. Acta Neurochir Suppl 2003;85:21–8.
4. Bejjani BP, Dormont D, Pidoux B, et al. Bilateral subthalamic stimulation for Parkinson's disease by using three-dimensional stereotactic magnetic resonance imaging and electrophysiological guidance. J Neurosurg 2000;92(4):615–25.
5. Starr PA, Christine CW, Theodosopoulos PV, et al. Implantation of deep brain stimulators into the subthalamic nucleus: technical approach and magnetic resonance imaging-verified lead locations. J Neurosurg 2002;97(2):370–87.
6. Carpentier A, McNichols RJ, Stafford RJ, et al. Real-time magnetic resonance-guided laser thermal therapy for focal metastatic brain tumors. Neurosurgery 2008; 63(1 Suppl 1):ONS21–8 [discussion: ONS28–9].
7. Merkle EM, Shonk JR, Zheng L, et al. MR imaging-guided radiofrequency thermal ablation in the porcine brain at 0.2 T. Eur Radiol 2001;11(5):884–92.
8. Lee MW, De Salles AA, Frighetto L, et al. Deep brain stimulation in intraoperative MRI environment—comparison of imaging techniques and electrode fixation methods. Minim Invasive Neurosurg 2005;48(1):1–6.
9. Martin AJ, Larson PS, Ostrem JL, et al. Placement of deep brain stimulator electrodes using real-time

high-field interventional magnetic resonance imaging. Magn Reson Med 2005;54(5):1107–14.

10. Liu H, Hall WA, Truwit CL. Neuronavigation in interventional MR imaging. Prospective stereotaxy. Neuroimaging Clin N Am 2001;11(4):695–704.

11. Truwit CL, Liu H. Prospective stereotaxy: a novel method of trajectory alignment using real-time image guidance. J Magn Reson Imaging 2001; 13(3):452–7.

12. Martin AJ, Hall WA, Roark C, et al. Minimally invasive precision brain access using prospective stereotaxy and a trajectory guide. J Magn Reson Imaging 2008; 27(4):737–43.

13. Moche M, Trampel R, Kahn T, et al. Navigation concepts for MR image-guided interventions. J Magn Reson Imaging 2008;27(2):276–91.

14. Yutzy SR, Duerk JL. Pulse sequences and system interfaces for interventional and real-time MRI. J Magn Reson Imaging 2008;27(2):267–75.

15. Guttman MA, Ozturk C, Raval AN, et al. Interventional cardiovascular procedures guided by real-time MR imaging: an interactive interface using multiple slices,

adaptive projection modes and live 3D renderings. J Magn Reson Imaging 2007;26(6):1429–35.

16. Maurer CR Jr, Hill DL, Martin AJ, et al. Investigation of intraoperative brain deformation using a 1.5-T interventional MR system: preliminary results. IEEE Trans Med Imaging 1998;17(5):817–25.

17. Arbel T, Morandi X, Comeau RM, et al. Automatic non-linear MRI-ultrasound registration for the correction of intra-operative brain deformations. Comput Aided Surg 2004;9(4):123–36.

18. Rachinger J, von Keller B, Ganslandt O, et al. Application accuracy of automatic registration in frameless stereotaxy. Stereotact Funct Neurosurg 2006; 84(2-3):109–17.

19. Pandya A, Siadat MR, Auner G. Design, implementation and accuracy of a prototype for medical augmented reality. Comput Aided Surg 2005;10(1): 23–35.

20. Wacker FK, Vogt S, Khamene A, et al. An augmented reality system for MR image-guided needle biopsy: initial results in a swine model. Radiology 2006;238(2):497–504.

# Devices for Targeting the Needle

Carol J. Barbre, BS

## KEYWORDS

- Stereotactic • Frameless stereotaxy • Smart frame
- Image-guided surgery • Interventional MRI

Stereotactic (also stereotaxy), literally translated from Greek and Latin, means "to touch in three dimensions" (stereo = three dimensions; tactic = to touch). In the medical sense, the term is defined as "a precise method of identifying nonvisualized anatomic structures by use of three-dimensional coordinates."[1] The three-dimensional space is generally defined by the X, Y, and Z Cartesian coordinate system (**Fig. 1**).

The most definitive description of the principles and device for stereotactic surgery is usually credited to Robert Henry Clarke and Victory Horsley, in their detailing and design of an apparatus to study cerebellar function in the monkey. In 1906, they wrote that "by this means every cubic millimeter of the brain could be studied and recorded."[2] A more complete description of the stereotactic instrument, atlas, and methods was reported in their classic paper of 1908. The Horsley-Clarke device was based on the reproducibility of the relationships between landmarks on the skull (external auditory canals, inferior orbital rims, midline) and anatomic structures within the brain of the experimental animal. The cranial fixation points established the baselines of a three-dimensional Cartesian stereotactic coordinate system.[2]

In neurosurgery the three-dimensional coordinate system is used by targeting devices to establish a trajectory path from a fixed point outside the brain to a specific point inside the brain. These targeting devices can be grouped into two distinct categories: (1) frame based, and (2) frameless. In general terms, the three-dimensional coordinate system is integrated in the frame-based system, whereas frameless devices rely on a separate, nonintegrated coordinate system. In the modern surgical era, it is difficult to separate the targeting device from surgical planning software, because the targeting device provides the link between preoperative planning and intraoperative navigation.

## DEVICE TYPE DESCRIPTION
### Frame-based Devices

Frame-based stereotactic devices are rigid external structures securely attached to the head using skull pins. The frame has four main functions: (1) to enable registration of image space to physical space; (2) to establish the three-dimensional X, Y, Z coordinate system; (3) to serve as the mechanism that holds and guides the surgical instrument; and (4) to maintain the patient's head in a fixed position relative to the coordinate system. Registration of image space to physical space is accomplished by way of fiducial markers that are part of the frame base. In clinical practice, before surgery, images are taken with the frame mounted to the patient's head. The fiducial markers are then used to coregister the patient to the preoperative images. This coregistration establishes the link for the surgical planning software to create a trajectory that will guide instruments by way of the frame's coordinate system.

The surgical planning software calculates the coordinates of the target and allows the user to create a trajectory to reach the target. Surgical instruments are then mounted to the frame and guided along the established trajectory. The two most widely used frame-based devices are the Leksell Stereotactic System (Elekta, Stockholm,

SurgiVision, Inc., 5 Musick, Irvine, CA 92618, USA
*E-mail address:* cbarbre@surgivision.com

Neurosurg Clin N Am 20 (2009) 187–191
doi:10.1016/j.nec.2009.04.006
1042-3680/09/$ – see front matter © 2009 Elsevier Inc. All rights reserved.

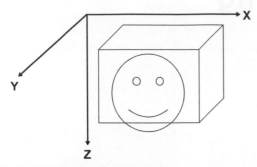

**Fig. 1.** Cartesian coordinate system.

Sweden) and the CRW Stereotactic System (Integra Radionics, Burlington, Massachusetts).

## Leksell Frame

The Leksell frame, developed in the late 1940s by Dr. Lars Leksell, is still in use today (**Fig. 2**). The frame is based on the center-of-arc principle, and the basic components are the Cartesian coordinate frame and a semicircular arc. The frame provides freedom of choice in trajectory and entry point selection such that all entry points provide a trajectory that passes through the center of the arc.

Frame fixation to the patient's head is achieved with adjustable fixation posts and screws. The frame consists of posterior, left-side, and right-side bars, which are permanently connected and cannot be disassembled. The anterior bar of the frame is exchangeable so that differently shaped pieces can be used, which provides flexibility in terms of access to the patient's nose and mouth and frame positioning. Markings are engraved on the frame and arc components for the X, Y, and Z coordinates. After the frame is fixed to the patient's head, the arc is attached to the frame

(**Fig. 3**). The arc is positioned according to the target's previously calculated X, Y, and Z coordinates so that the center of the arc coincides with the selected brain target. Because of the freedom of choice for the entry point, the area of interest can be targeted from any position on the arc.

## CRW Frame

Introduced in 1979, the CRW frame consists of a separate frame base and arc system (**Fig. 4**). The frame is fixed to the patient's head using four self-penetrating screws. It is not an arc-centered system, which is the major distinction between the CRW and Leksell frames. Patient and surgical site access is accomplished with various tools. A 30° offset probe holder gives unobstructed access to the surgical site, head ring extenders shift the scannable volume for deep tumors, and a removable anterior plate provides patient comfort and airway access. Submillimeter settings are achieved with vernier scales at each arc and target setting (**Fig. 5**). The system can be configured as a basic CT-only system, a CT/MR scanner-dependent system, or a CT/MR scanner-independent system.

## First Generation Frameless System

As an alternative to the frame-based system, the burr hole–mounted system was developed. This type of system offered less flexibility in trajectory and entry point selection because it had only two angular degrees of freedom and a depth stop adjustment. The early burr hole–mounted systems were not popular because they required significant mathematical calculations and were prone to angular errors. Often the target was assessed intraoperatively by taking multiple radiographs to determine position and then making any

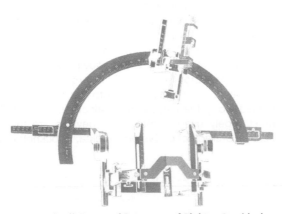

**Fig. 2.** Leksell Frame. (*Courtesy of* Elekta, Stockholm, Sweden; with permission.)

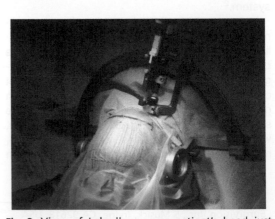

**Fig. 3.** View of Leksell arc over patient's head just before scalp incision. (*Courtesy of* D. Lim, MD, PhD, San Francisco, CA.)

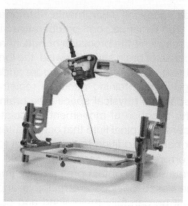

**Fig. 4.** CRW Stereotactic System. (*Courtesy of* Integra Radionics, Burlington, MA; with permission.)

necessary trajectory adjustments on the frame. This process, however, resulted in multiple penetrations of the brain.

## Modern Day Frameless Devices

The current generation of frameless stereotactic devices is much smaller than their frame-based counterparts. They attach directly over the planned entry point on the patient's skull. The frameless devices provide the mechanism that holds the surgical instruments and guides them along the prescribed trajectory. These devices, however, must rely on a separate system of reference or fiducial markers because they lack the frame that performs this function on the frame-based systems. Fiducial markers are therefore attached directly to the scalp or skull to provide the reference points to register the patient's position in physical space. The frame and other instruments are in turn registered by the surgical planning computer through a method of recognition or localization. One such method is an optical tracking system, whereby an array of cameras is used to locate the fiducials and instruments and transmit information to the surgical planning computer.

The two frameless systems that are most commonly used are the NexFrame (Medtronic, Minneapolis, Minnesota) and the StarFix microTargeting Platform (FHC, Bowdoinham, Maine). The NexFrame is a plastic apparatus that mounts around the burr hole (**Fig. 6**). Its upper component rotates and translates, providing the ability to aim the device within a 50-degree arc. The NexFrame was designed specifically for deep brain stimulation placement and works with most common micropositioners, including one specifically designed for it. An optical tracking system in combination with bone-implanted fiducials allows the system to be registered with a surgical navigation system. The surgeon can therefore manipulate the device in real time to aim it at the desired target while watching reconstructed MR images (**Fig. 7**). This device has been successfully implemented in intraoperative MRI (iMRI) for deep brain stimulation surgery.[3,4]

The StarFix is a skull-mounted tripod-like device that is custom manufactured in advance according to a three-dimensional model of the patient's skull based on presurgical imaging. A high-resolution

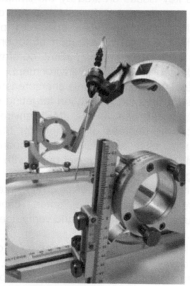

**Fig. 5.** CRW Stereotactic showing coordinate system's markings. (*Courtesy of* Integra Radionics, Burlington, MA; with permission.)

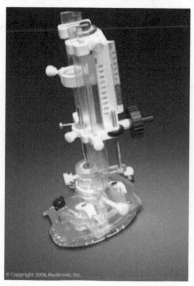

**Fig. 6.** NexFrame and NexDrive. (*Courtesy of* Medtronic, Inc., Minneapolis, MN; with permission.)

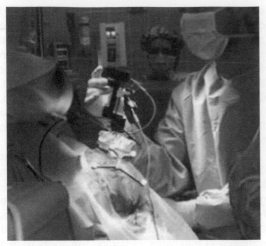

**Fig. 7.** View of the NexFrame during DBS placement. (*Courtesy of* P. Larson, MD, San Francisco, CA.)

CT of the patient is obtained several days before surgery, and the surgeon plans the surgery in advance, including target selection, entry point, and trajectory. The CT and plan are then transmitted to a manufacturing facility, which custom makes the device and ships it to the surgical center. On the day of surgery, the StarFix is attached to the skull at predetermined attachment points and is already aimed at the predesignated target (**Fig. 8**). There is therefore no need for an optical tracking or surgical navigation system.[4,5]

## LIMITATIONS OF CURRENT TARGETING DEVICES

Today's functional neurosurgery procedures demand submillimetric accuracy. Both frame-based and frameless devices rely on three-dimensional reference systems and preoperative images

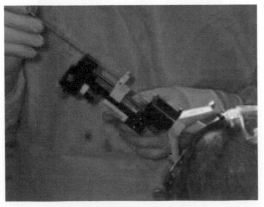

**Fig. 8.** StarFix microTargeting Platform. (*Courtesy of* FHC, Inc., Bowdoin, MF; with permission.)

to guide surgical instruments intraoperatively (**Table 1**). Reliance on preoperative images, though, may limit the precision of patient registration because of brain shift. Likewise, the long duration of the current surgical procedure adds to the challenge of maintaining accurate registration of image space to physical space. The brain generally shifts because of movement associated with loss of cerebral spinal fluid that occurs after drilling the burr hole. In addition to the potential for registration errors, current targeting devices require a separate scan to obtain preoperative images.

Frame-based devices are reusable and therefore must be carefully maintained and calibrated to obtain optimum performance. Accuracy of frame-based systems depends in large part on the physical structure of the frame. Although frameless devices may be more comfortable for the patient than their frame-based counterparts (both types of devices are generally used on awake patients), the complexity of use of these frameless devices may have limited the rate of adoption. Frameless devices are disposable, designed for a single patient's use, so calibration is less of an issue. Given that frameless devices rely on an independent, nonintegrated X, Y, Z coordinate system, their accuracy relies on the accuracy of the optical tracking systems or other locating methods.

## DEVICES OF THE FUTURE
### Optimal Features of a Targeting Device

The next generation of targeting devices needs to address key issues created by the limitations of today's systems: need for a preoperative scan, errors in registering image space to physical space, lack of target visualization intraoperatively, lengthy procedure times, patient comfort, and poor adaptability to the MR environment.

Some of the more desirable characteristics and features for the next generation targeting device, particularly for use in the iMRI environment, include: large degrees of freedom for trajectory adjustment, ease and flexibility of mounting to the skull, motorized instrument guide with remote steering mechanisms, ability to create a parallel path with a high degree of flexibility, integrated software capabilities, and a "smart" cannula or guide tube that could detect and verify deep brain targets.

Development of the next generation of devices is underway, such as the adjustable, skull-mounted trajectory guide and software platform in development at SurgiVision. This system, called ClearPoint (SurgiVision Inc., Irvine, California), is a real-time MRI-guided neuro intervention system.

**Table 1**
**Comparison of targeting devices**

|  | Frame Based | Frameless | Smart Frames |
|---|---|---|---|
| Use of preoperative imaging | Yes | Yes | None |
| Preoperative skull-mounted fiducial markers | Yes (part of frame) | Yes | None |
| Potential for registration errors | Yes | Yes | Minimal |
| Ability to account for brain shift | None | None | Yes |

The ClearPoint trajectory guide is different from the frame-based and frameless devices available today; it could be called a "smart frame." The trajectory guide contains integrated, software-detectable fiducial markers. The guide is actively linked to MRI space, eliminating the need for traditional fiducial-based registration. In essence, physical space and image space now become one—MR space.

The ClearPoint system includes the MR-readable frame, an MR-readable marking grid that identifies the optimal location of the burr hole, and proprietary software that provides real-time trajectory guidance. A key feature of the software is that it streams raw DICOM MR data from multiple manufacturers' scanning platforms, providing consistency in the look and feel of the procedure. The frame is designed for single use and is small enough to allow for two frames to be mounted simultaneously for bilateral procedures. It is mounted on the skull directly over the burr hole and has four control knobs to remotely adjust the instrument's trajectory under MR guidance.

## SUMMARY

Targeting devices for neurosurgery have evolved since their introduction last century, and the application of surgical planning software has helped to facilitate improvements in neurosurgical techniques. The inability to visualize the target in real time remains a limiting factor for traditional targeting devices, however. A targeting device that works in combination with MRI would resolve many of the challenges of today's devices.

## REFERENCES

1. Stedman's Medical Dictionary, 27th edition. p. 1697.
2. Cyber museum of neurosurgery. Development of experimental stereotactic systems (1873–1932). Available at: http://www.neurosurgery.org/Cybermuseum/ stereotactichall/stereoarticle.html. Accessed October 17, 2008.
3. Holloway KL, Gaede SE, Starr PA, et al. Frameless stereotaxy using bone fiducials markers for deep brain stimulation. J Neurosurg 2005;103:404–13.
4. Larson Paul S, et al. Technical alternatives in performing deep brain stimulator implantation. In: Tarsy Daniel, Vitek Jerrold L, Starr Philip A, editors. Deep brain stimulation in neurological and psychiatric disorders. Totowa (NJ): Humana Press; 2008. p. 101.
5. Fitzpatrick JM, Konrad PE, Nickele C, et al. Accuracy of customized miniature stereotactic platforms. Stereotact Funct Neurosurg 2005;83:25–31.

# The Development of Robotics for Interventional MRI

Shelly Lwu, MD, MSc[a], Garnette R. Sutherland, MD[a,b],*

**KEYWORDS**
- Neurosurgery • Robotics • Intraoperative MRI
- NeuroArm • Human machine interface

Progress in neurosurgery has, to a large extent, paralleled advances in technology. With the introduction of the operating microscope and microsurgical technique, surgical corridors became increasingly narrow, accelerating the development of complimentary instrumentation.[1] The inventions of CT and MRI provided unprecedented preoperative lesion localization, allowing neurosurgeons to plan more precisely targeted approaches.[2–5] These imaging techniques, in addition to enabling lesion localization, gave clinicians better insight into diagnosis prior to surgery. The 1990s saw the introduction and widespread use of computer-based image guidance systems that allowed intraoperative surgical navigation based on preoperative images. Due mainly to the problem of brain shift associated with craniotomy and surgical dissection, CT and MRI technologies were brought into the operating room and integrated with neurosurgery.[6–10] The integration of robotic technology into surgical procedure represents the culmination of a logical progression that takes full advantage of these innovations. Robotic technology offers the potential for increased precision and accuracy and, when coupled with ongoing advances in neuroscience and the integrative and executive capacity of the human brain, provides an unparalleled opportunity to improve neurosurgical outcome.

This article presents a brief review of the evolution of neurosurgical robots, the challenges associated with the development of a magnetic resonance (MR)–compatible image-guided robot, and an overview of the manufacture, integration, and initial clinical experiences of such a robot, neuroArm.

## EVOLUTION OF THE NEUROSURGICAL ROBOT

The first neurosurgical robots performed only simple, well-defined tasks. One of these was the Programmable Universal Machine for Assembly (PUMA; Advance Research and Robotics, Oxford, Connecticut), an industrial robot adapted for neurosurgery.[11] It had a single arm with six degrees of freedom (DOF). With a personal computer, the arm could be programmed to move in line with the planned trajectory or be moved passively into position. Preoperative CT images, taken with the Brown-Roberts-Wells head frame, were used to determine stereotactic coordinates and to provide three-dimensional (3D) reconstructions of the target lesion and surrounding anatomical structures in relation to the probe. In 1991, Drake and colleagues[12] reported the successful application of the PUMA 200 robot as a retractor holder in the resections of thalamic astrocytomas in six children (**Fig. 1**). Safety concerns with regards to the use of an industrial robot in surgery halted further development of PUMA for applications related to neurosurgery.

NeuroMate (Integrated Surgical Systems, Davis, California), developed specifically for neurosurgery, was intended for stereotactic procedures with image guidance.[13] NeuroMate has a single

[a] Department of Clinical Neurosciences, University of Calgary, 1403 29th street NW, Calgary, Alberta T2N 2T9, Canada
[b] Seaman Family MR Research Centre, University of Calgary, 1403 29th street NW, Calgary, Alberta T2N 2T9, Canada
* Corresponding author.
*E-mail address:* garnette@ucalgary.ca (G.R. Sutherland).

Neurosurg Clin N Am 20 (2009) 193–206
doi:10.1016/j.nec.2009.04.011

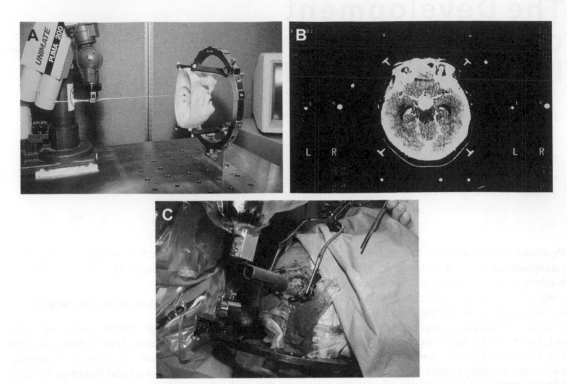

**Fig. 1.** The PUMA 200 is a six-DOF manipulator capable of moving at a peak velocity of 1 m/s while carrying a payload of 1 kg. (*A*) The PUMA 200 arm directs a probe towards the planned target in a skull. (*B*) A preoperative CT scan taken with the Brown-Roberts-Wells stereotactic frame shows a thalamic astrocytoma. Stereotactic coordinates are calculated from the preoperative imaging. (*C*) The PUMA arm, gripping a retractor, moves into position in the surgical field. (*Courtesy of* James Drake, MD, University of Toronto, Canada.)

arm with five DOF and is capable of gripping or stabilizing surgical instruments, such as cannulas and biopsy needles (**Fig. 2**). Using preoperative CT or MRI, the target lesion and trajectory are defined at the computer workstation and the robot arm is commanded into position. NeuroMate is compatible with both frame-based and frameless stereotaxy; the frameless mode uses an ultrasound registration system. NeuroMate, the first robot approved by the Food and Drug Administration for use in stereotactic neurosurgical procedures, has been used for tumor biopsies and various functional procedures, including electrode placement for deep brain stimulation.[14]

Evolution 1 (Universal Robot Systems, Schwerin, Germany) was designed to enhance positional accuracy and precision of movement in microsurgical and neuroendoscopic procedures. Evolution 1, a hexapod robot with six DOF,[15] operates using high-precision linear axes and joints and has an absolute positional accuracy of 20 μm and motion resolution of 1 μm while carrying payloads of up to 50 kg. The mobile platform can accommodate a variety of surgical instruments, including an endoscope. During surgery, the surgeon at the

workstation uses a joystick to direct the robot with the aid of neuronavigation and preoperative MRI. Evolution 1 has been used in the positioning and maneuvering of ventriculoscopes in neuroendoscopy.[15] Functioning in a similar role in endoscopic transsphenoidal resections of pituitary adenomas, Evolution 1 enables surgeons to operate using two instruments simultaneously.[16]

The integration of intraoperative image guidance with neurosurgical robots followed. Minerva (University of Lausanne, Switzerland),[17] a robot with a five-DOF arm, was designed to perform stereotactic neurosurgical procedures within the CT scanner. Minerva occupied a position at the head of the operating table, behind the CT scanner, so that its arm could work within the gantry. Successive CT image acquisition during the procedure updated the instrument position in near real-time, thus providing intraoperative image guidance. The system automated the tasks of making skin incisions, drilling bone, performing dural perforations, and manipulating probes.[18] Applications of Minerva in stereotactic tumor biopsies were successful.[17,18] Even so, the project was discontinued, apparently because of CT imaging

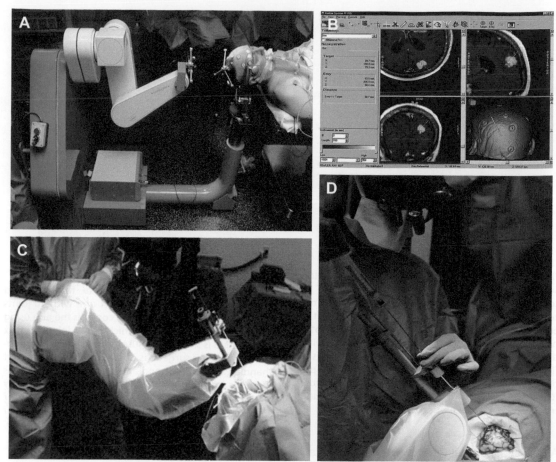

**Fig. 2.** NeuroMate is a five-DOF manipulator designed to assist with stereotactic neurosurgical procedures in both frame-based and frameless modes. (*A*) Registration of the NeuroMate arm to the patient using a frameless ultrasound registration system. (*B*) Screenshot of the neuronavigation system demonstrating the target lesion in three planes on the preoperative MRI, as well as the planned trajectory in a 3D reconstruction. (*C*) The NeuroMate arm is positioned in the surgical field in line with the planned trajectory and in preparation for the biopsy. (*D*) The neurosurgeon performs the frameless stereotactic biopsy with NeuroMate acting in the role of the assistant, stabilizing the biopsy cannula. (*Courtesy of* Qing Hang Li, MD, PhD, Wayne State University, Detroit, MI.)

that was only one-dimensional and because of high radiation exposure to the patient.

Several MR-compatible robot projects are in development. Harvard Medical School and the Surgical Planning Laboratory of Brigham and Women's Hospital (Boston, Massachusetts) collaborated with the Surgical Assist Technology Group of the Agency of Industrial Science and Technology (Tsukuba, Japan) to develop a robot that could work within an intraoperative MRI system based on a 0.5-T double-donut magnet (Signa SP/i; General Electric, Milwaukee, Wisconsin) (**Fig. 3**).[19] The body of the robot and its actuators are located above the neurosurgeon's head and the end effector is attached to the body of the robot by two long rigid arms. The end effector has five DOF and functions as an aid for the manual insertion of probes in stereotactic procedures.

The Mechatronics Laboratory at the University of Tokyo, Japan, uses a different design concept. Also intended for stereotactic neurosurgery, the MR-compatible needle position manipulator operates within the 60-cm gradient aperture of a diagnostic MR system.[20] The manipulator and the six-DOF stereotactic frame to which it is mounted are attached to the scanner bed to ensure precision. The neurosurgeon controls the manipulator from a personal computer located in an adjacent room.

Robots with greater dexterity and enhanced tool manipulation abilities are being developed for microsurgery. Robot-Assisted Microsurgery System (RAMS; National Aeronautic and Space

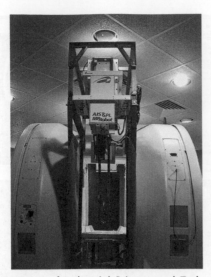

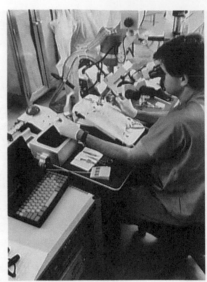

**Fig. 3.** Agency of Industrial Science and Technology/ Surgical Planning Laboratory MR Robot. This MR-compatible robot is mounted at the top of a horizontal field open-gantry double-donut magnet. Its end effector is attached to the body of the robot via two long rigid arms. The neurosurgeon stands within the air gap of the double-donut magnet and uses the five-DOF end effector as an aid for the precise positioning of probes during stereotactic procedures. (*Courtesy of* Kiyoyuki Chinzei, PhD, Agency of Industrial Science and Technology, Tsukuba, Japan.)

**Fig. 4.** RAMS, a system designed for enhanced dexterity, has a single slave robot arm with 10 joints and six DOF. The neurosurgeon controls the arm using the master input handle, which has 8 joints and six DOF. RAMS is shown in a surgical setup. Under microscopic view, the surgeon is operating the master input handle with his left hand and using a pair of forceps with his right hand to work on a rat in a laboratory setting. The laptop computer to the left is used for the configuration of system parameters. (*Courtesy of* Peter D. Le Roux, MD, University of Pennsylvania, Philadelphia, PA.)

Administration's Jet Propulsion Laboratory, Pasadena, California, and MicroDexterity Systems Inc., Memphis, Tennessee) has a single slave robot arm with 10 joints and six DOF. The neurosurgeon controls the arm using the master input handle with 8 joints and six DOF (**Fig. 4**).[21] The neurosurgeon manipulates the master input handle in the same manner as a conventional surgical instrument. The entire system, under computer control, employs a laptop computer with graphical user interface for the configuration of system parameters. Features for enhancement of surgical performance have been incorporated into RAMS, including force scaling, motion scaling, and tremor filtering. Force feedback is not included in the system. While feasibility studies have demonstrated that RAMS is capable of functioning as the nondominant hand in microvascular anastomosis and knot-tying exercises, RAMS is not capable of holding needles or performing suturing.

The Steady Hand robotics system (Johns Hopkins University, Baltimore, Maryland) also enhances surgical performance without taking the neurosurgeon away from the operating table. The surgeon manipulates tools held by the Steady Hand robot (**Fig. 5**).[22,23] The system has incorporated tremor filters, motion scaling, and force

sensors to provide smooth and tremor-free tissue manipulation with precision and a delicate touch.

NeuRobot (Shinshu University School of Medicine, Matsumoto, Japan) is a robotic system intended for minimally invasive microsurgery.[24] NeuRobot has one long, thin manipulator arm, which houses a rigid 3D endoscope and three micromanipulators. Each micromanipulator has three DOF (**Fig. 6**). Operating under master-slave command, each micromanipulator has a corresponding hand controller at the workstation. During surgery, the operator manipulates the joysticks at the remote workstation while wearing polarizing glasses and watching the display monitor. NeuRobot has been used successfully in both preclinical and clinical trials.[24,25] To demonstrate the feasibility in telesurgery, clinicians have successfully performed surgery in an animal model in a hospital 40 km away from the workstation.[26]

## UNIQUE CHALLENGES TO THE DEVELOPMENT OF A MAGNETIC RESONANCE–COMPATIBLE ROBOT

Formidable challenges await anyone trying to develop a neurosurgical robot capable of

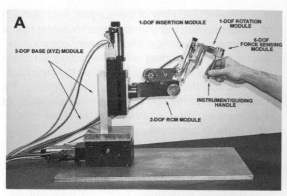

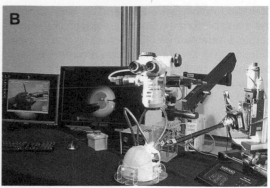

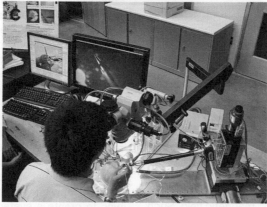

**Fig. 5.** The Steady Hand robot is a manipulator designed to enhance the surgeon's performance. The surgeon manipulates the surgical instrument gripped by the Steady Hand robot. (*A*) A second-generation Steady Hand robot is shown with the surgeon's hand holding the instrument-guiding handle. (*B*) The current surgical workstation consists of the third-generation Steady Hand robot, a video microscope, a monitor displaying a two-dimensional view from the microscope, and a second monitor displaying system configuration. (*C*) The Steady Hand robot being used in a phantom study. (*Courtesy of* Russell Taylor, PhD, Johns Hopkins University, Baltimore, MD; with permission.)

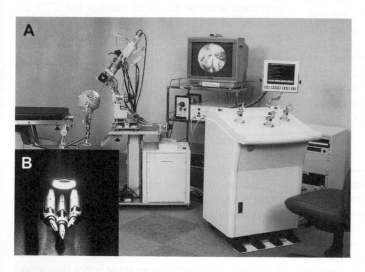

**Fig. 6.** NeuRobot is a system designed for minimally invasive microsurgery. (*A*) The slave manipulator arm is in position at the head of the operating table. The workstation, with the three master hand controllers, and the display monitor can be placed within the operating room or located remotely. (*B*) The end of the manipulator arm houses three micromanipulators and a rigid 3D endoscope. All three of the micromanipulators are displayed with the microforceps attachments, each with a payload of 60 g. The microforceps can be substituted for laser tips, scalpels, and dissectors as needed during surgery. Note the three hand controllers at the workstation correspond to the three micromanipulators. (*Fig. 5A courtesy of* Kazuhiro Hongo, MD, Shinshu University School of Medicine, Matsumoto, Japan. *Fig. 5B from* Koyama J, Hongo K, Kakizawa Y, et al. Endoscopic telerobotics for neurosurgery: preliminary study for optimal distance between an object lens and a target. Neurological Research 2002;24:374; with permission.)

operating within an intraoperative MRI environment and performing both stereotactic and microsurgical procedures. First, such a robot must function in a sensoryimmersive environment and be able to replicate the surgical experience for the neurosurgeon. Second, the robot must be designed so that it can be integrated seamlessly into the preexisting surgical process in a manner safe for both the patient and the surgical team. Third, the robot must accommodate telecapability so the workstation can be positioned outside the magnetic field of the MRI system.

### Magnetic Resonance Compatibility

MR compatibility significantly influences robot design and material selection. The ideal MR-compatible robot should not degrade MRI quality. Likewise, the electromagnetic field should not disturb the robot's performance. Magnetic susceptibility and electrical conductivity, features that determine MR compatibility, make it particularly difficult to develop suitable actuators and force sensors.[27] While the use of ferromagnetic materials within an MR environment poses an obvious safety concern, consideration must also be given to induced eddy currents in the conducting materials within a working magnetic field. Such currents can result in thermal and electrical burns to the patient. Plastic polymers, such as polyether-etherketone, polyoxymethylene, and polyethylene terephthalate, and ceramics have negligible magnetic susceptibility and therefore are ideal for the construction of an MR-compatible robot.[28] These materials are relatively MR invisible. They have little effect on signal-to-noise ratio, and would not be seen within the imaging volume. Other materials that have been used for robotic components include aluminum, titanium, glass, and beryllium-copper. While these materials are MR compatible, they do affect signal-to-noise ratio and produce susceptibility artifacts if seen within the imaging volume.[28] Payload and speed requirements make titanium a favored construction material.

### Human-machine Interface

With the primary neurosurgeon no longer at the surgical site, the system requires technology to re-create the surgical site and the elements of surgical dissection at a remote workstation.[29,30] A human-machine interface with multiple sensory inputs and outputs is necessary to re-create the visual, audio, and tactile feedback of the surgical environment. Each sensory element is considered important for the successful blending of machine technology with human ability. The surgeon needs

the stereoscopic view of the surgical field through the microscope, the sound of manipulating tissue of varying consistency, and two-way communication with the operating room personnel. Of more importance and perhaps essential, the neurosurgeon needs the sense of touch and position for delicate tissue manipulation. The reproduction of tactile sensibility is and remains the most difficult challenge to surmount.

### Stereotactic Procedures and Microsurgery

No previous neurosurgical robot has included the capability of both stereotaxy and microsurgery. To represent the primary surgeon at the surgical site during microsurgery, the robot should have at least two manipulators to mimic the surgeon's two arms. Interactions with operating room personnel should remain similar to those employed in established surgical routines for minimal disruption of surgical rhythm. Such interactions include positioning the manipulators into the surgical field so as not to interfere with tool exchange and the activities of the assistant surgeon and scrub nurse. For stereotaxy, the manipulator needs to be able to work inside the gradient aperture of the magnet. The challenge was to create a system that could be adaptable to both sterotaxy and microsurgery.

### Safety

Safety is always a concern when there is interaction between people and machines. If stereotactic procedures are to be performed within the magnet gantry, then access to the anesthetized patient is restricted and the ability to monitor the ECG ST segment during imaging is limited. This means that this technology has limited applications to patients with significant cardiac disease. In addition, imaging has the potential to affect robotic encoders, necessitating gating image acquisition to robotic movement. The recent introduction of optical encoders may well circumvent this need. Even if a robot is operating under master-slave control, encoder malfunction could result in unintended movement with potential injury. The extent of movement depends on how fast the system recognizes the malfunction and stops further movement. Safety analysis for any robotic system is mandatory prior to widespread clinical use.

### NEUROARM IN DEPTH

NeuroArm is the MR-compatible robot developed from a collaboration between MacDonald Dettweiler and Associates (Brampton, Ontario, Canada) and the Seaman Family MR Research

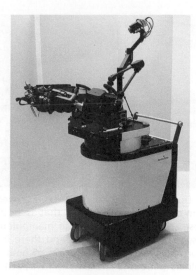

**Fig. 7.** NeuroArm's two manipulators, digitizing arm, and field camera are mounted on an adjustable base. NeuroArm's two manipulators mimic the actions of the neurosurgeon. Each manipulator has seven DOF.

Centre at the University of Calgary, Foothills Medical Center (Calgary, Alberta, Canada).[29–32] NeuroArm is intended for stereotactic surgery within the bore of the magnet and microsurgery outside the magnet.

## Robot

NeuroArm consists of two manipulator arms, one digitizing arm, and a field camera mounted on an adjustable mobile base (**Fig. 7**). The two manipulators mimic the two arms of the primary neurosurgeon. Each manipulator has seven DOF, including one DOF for tool actuation. Operating under a master-slave control system, the manipulators replicate the surgeon's movements of the

handcontrollers at the workstation. During surgery, after the perioperative images have been obtained, the robot is positioned next to the operating room table, where the primary neurosurgeon would stand, and locked in place using a wheel brake. A counter-balance mechanism, based on elevator design, allows easy adjustment of the base height.

For MR compatibility, the manipulators are made from titanium and two plastic polymers, polyetheretherketone and polyoxymethylene (**Fig. 8**). The end effector of each manipulator contains custom-made titanium multiaxis force and torque sensors (ATI Industrial Automation, Apex, North Carolina), located directly between the tool and the end effector. These force sensors provide haptic feedback to the hand controllers at the workstation in three translational DOF. The use of two of these high-resolution strain gauge sensors allows better distinction of the forces associated with tool actuation from gravity.

Each end effector accommodates a specially designed set of MR-compatible tools. Based on standard surgical instruments currently in use, modifications were made so the instruments can be adapted to and actuated by the robot end effectors. They include bipolar forceps, needle drivers, suction devices, biopsy forceps, microscissors, and microdissectors. While the prototype tools were based on titanium to withstand gas and autoclave sterilization, designers intend to convert the biopsy and implantation tools to ceramics. Ceramics are ideal because they have minimal effect on imaging signals regardless of the strength of the magnetic field.[28]

A partially automated tool exchange occurs at the end effector to mimic the surgeon-nurse interaction. To ensure minimal disruption to established surgical processes, the neuroArm is designed to accommodate tool exchange in 2 to

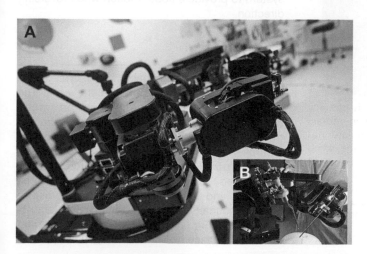

**Fig. 8.** (*A*) NeuroArm's two manipulators are made from MR-compatible materials: titanium, polyetheretherketone, and polyoxymethylene. (*B*) Custom-made titanium multiaxis force and torque sensors are located between the tool and the end effector. The sensors assist in replicating the tactile experience of surgery by providing haptic feedback to the hand controllers at the workstation in three translational DOF.

3 seconds. At the command of the surgeon, the manipulator moves to a predetermined tool exchange site, where the instrument is exchanged manually by the scrub nurse (**Fig. 9**). The tool holder has a functional and simple design for rapid tool exchange. For safety, the tool is scanned with a bar scanner and the surgeon at the workstation is provided with verbal confirmation that the desired tool has been inserted. In the event of system failure, the tool can be removed manually and the manipulator can be moved outside the surgical field. The speed and payload requirements of the manipulators were determined based on the maximum amount of time allowable during surgery to perform tool exchange with the heaviest tool expected, accelerating to 200 mm/s during tool exchange while carrying a payload of 500 g.

Custom drapes were designed to maintain sterility (**Fig. 10**). Tool holders are sterilized and designed to penetrate the drape while maintaining sterility. Because the drapes are clear, movements and joint position can be seen throughout surgery. The drapes are loose to allow heat dissipation and prevent constriction of motion. Appropriate drapes are essential to allow safe integration of machine technology into surgical processes.

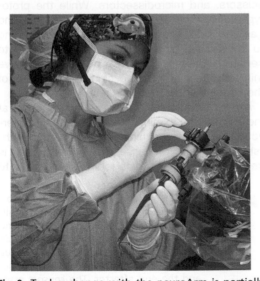

**Fig. 9.** Tool exchange with the neuroArm is partially automated to mimic the usual nurse-surgeon interaction in the operating room. Once the manipulator has moved into position for tool exchange, the scrub nurse manually exchanges the surgical instrument at the request of the surgeon. The speed and payload capabilities of the manipulators (accelerating to 200 mm/s during tool exchange while carrying a payload of 500 g), combined with the straightforward design of the tool holder, make it possible for the nurse to change tools in 10 to 20 seconds.

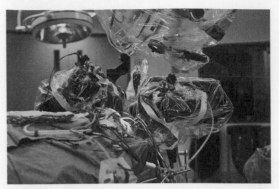

**Fig. 10.** During surgery, neuroArm is covered in a custom-designed sterile drape that is both clear and loose. The movements of the manipulators are clearly seen through the drapes and there is ample room for movement and dissipation of heat. Sterile tool holders penetrate the drapes to attach to the end effectors.

All of neuroArm's high-precision gears are made of titanium for MR compatibility. The ultrasonic piezoelectric actuators (Nanomotion, Yokneam, Israel) have an average lifespan of 20,000 hours and a resolution of 1 nm. The actuators brake if power is lost, an additional safety feature. The shoulder and wrist joints each require three motors to meet the high torque requirements. There are two additional motors for the wrist pitch joint. The heat generated from running neuroArm is conducted to the titanium housings and additional heat sinks. The input and output of each joint is provided by sine/cosine rotary electric encoders (Netzr Precision Motion Sensor, Misgav, Israel), which offer an accuracy of 0.01°. As an added benefit, the encoders retain positional information when powered off for intraoperative imaging. As an additional safety feature, antibacklash mechanics have been incorporated into the system to provide smooth motion when reversing direction.

### Workstation

As the neuroArm is telecapable, it is operated from a remote workstation in an adjacent room. The workstation is composed of a computer processor, two force-feedback hand controllers to maneuver the robot manipulators, a Spaceball 3D motion controller (3Dconnexion, Fremont, California) to manipulate the MRIs, four desk-mounted monitors (two video monitors and two touch-screen displays), and a binocular stereoscopic display unit, all mounted on an ergonomic height-adjustable table (**Fig. 11**). A multisensory human-machine interface has been developed to provide

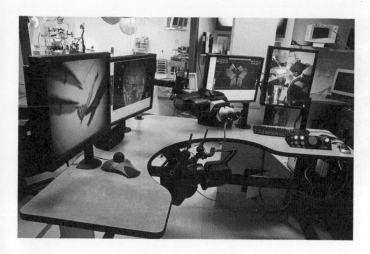

**Fig. 11.** The neuroArm workstation is in an adjacent room. The workstation consists of a computer processor, two force-feedback hand controllers to maneuver the robot manipulators, a Spaceball 3D motion controller to manipulate the MR images, four desk-mounted monitors (two video monitors and two touch-screen displays), and a binocular stereoscopic display unit, all mounted on an ergonomic height-adjustable table.

visual, audio, and tactile feedback to the neurosurgeon.

Visual feedback is provided primarily by the stereoscopic view of the surgical field through the binocular display unit and secondarily from the four monitors. Two high-definition cameras (Ikegami Tsushinki Co., Ltd., Tokyo, Japan) are mounted to the surgical microscope to provide images transmitted to two miniature full-color monitors (Rockwell Collins Inc., Cedar Rapids, Iowa) fitted within a binocular display unit, at 1000–television line horizontal resolution. The binocular display unit has the oculars from a standard operating microscope. The two video monitors display the field camera view and the single channel view from the left optic of the stereoscopic display unit, both at XGA (extended graphics array) 1024 × 768 resolution. The field camera is mounted above the manipulators during microsurgery and on the extension board to the operating table during stereotaxy. One touch-screen monitor displays two-dimensional (2D) and reconstructed 3D MRIs that can be manipulated for surgical planning and lesion localization. The surgeon can also add a virtual tool overlay to track the movement of the surgical tool in relation to the lesion and the brain in real time (**Fig. 12**). The MRIs can be manipulated using the touch screen or the Spaceball 3D motion controller. The second touch screen is a control panel, displaying neuroArm system status, commands, and settings with a virtual view of the robotic manipulators. A large-screen liquid crystal display monitor is mounted on the wall of the operating room showing a single-channel right optic view of the stereoscopic display for the surgical team.

Two-way communication between the personnel of the surgical team occurs via the DX200 Digital Wireless Intercom system (HM Electronics, Inc., Poway, California). A desk-mounted microphone and speakers at the workstation provide the operating surgeon with the ability to communicate with any individual or all of the surgical team together. In the operating room, headsets are worn by the surgical team, providing contact with the operating surgeon. In addition, a microphone mounted on the microscope transmits the sound of surgical dissection. Digital encryption and a frequency-hopping spread spectrum are used to block unauthorized eavesdropping. At a frequency of 2.4 GHz, there is no interference of the audio system transmission with the MRI as this is well outside of the MR frequency range.

Tactile feedback is provided by two customized Phantom haptic hand controllers (SensAble Technologies Inc., Woburn, Massachusetts), each with six DOF (**Fig. 13**). Each hand controller has a modified stylus designed to mimic

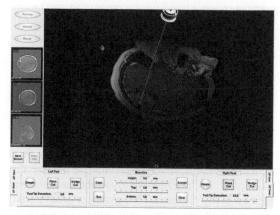

**Fig. 12.** The surgeon using the neuroArm has the option of adding a virtual tool overlay onto preoperatively acquired MR images to track the movement of the surgical instrument in relation to the target lesion and the brain in real time.

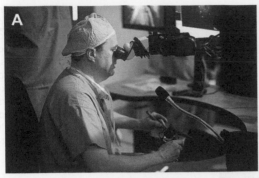
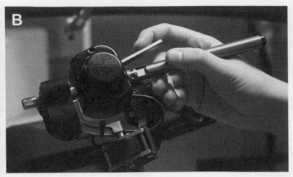

**Fig. 13.** (*A*) The primary surgeon operating the neuroArm uses two customized Phantom haptic hand controllers, each with six DOF, at the workstation. (*B*) Each hand controller has a modified stylus, which actuates the tool with an index finger–activated lever. A squeeze of the strain gauge switch by the thumb enables and disables the robot manipulators. (*Fig. 13A from* SensAble Technologies Inc., Woburn, MA; with permission.)

conventional hand-tool motion. The stylus has an index finger–activated lever for tool actuation and a strain gauge switch, which activates with a light squeeze of the thumb, for enabling and disabling the manipulators. Based on initial clinical experience, developers plan to convert activation control to a foot switch.

The haptic hand controllers were designed to replicate the surgeon-tool interface. Force sensors provide the neurosurgeon with real-time physical quantification of the deformation of brain tissue and, at the same time, accommodate force scaling, adjustments to limit the amount of force applied to the tissues. Force sensors and force scaling provide many potential benefits. The manipulation of brain tissue and cerebrovasculature has required a delicate touch that up until now has been virtually impossible to quantify. Now, with force sensors, the force applied by the neurosurgeon's hand can be measured and taught to neurosurgeons in training in a fashion that can be precisely copied and tested. Furthermore, force sensors give rise to the possibility that different force thresholds can be set for the different tissue types during microdissection. For example, in trying to dissect a tuberculum sella meningioma off an optic nerve, a much higher threshold can be set for the tumor in comparison to the optic nerve. Most importantly, neuroArm has the potential to augment the fine control of the force exerted by a skilled hand, which takes years to master. For example, to prevent inadvertent aneurysmal rupture in the dissection of vessels or brain parenchyma off an aneurysm, neuroArm can scale down a larger force exerted by the neurosurgeon at the hand controllers to a much smaller force than could be applied by a human hand. NeuroArm oould thus enable more effective performance

and teaching of the more technically challenging surgeries.

Similarly, motion scaling can translate a large displacement of the hand controller into a much smaller displacement of the surgical tool. Motion scaling has the ability to improve the spatial resolution of microdissection from millimeters to less than 50 μm. With further technological advances in imaging, microdissection could potentially be shifted from the present organ to the cellular level.

NeuroArm offers the option of tremor filtering to remove the physiological tremor of the human hand. Physiological tremor is an involuntary and almost sinusoidal movement, which can increase with age, fatigue, and caffeine consumption. Rather than actively suppressing the tremor, tremor filters offset the effects of the tremor by exerting an equal but opposite motion to that of the tool tip.[33] This capability adds to the complexity of the neuroArm's design because it means the tool must be able to sense its own motion and distinguish between the intended and unintended movements of the surgeon.[34] Tremor filtering has the ability to increase precision and decrease position error. Combined with force and motion scaling, tremor filtering has the potential of enhancing human surgical performance.

Using specially designed software, the neurosurgeon can incorporate an additional safety feature into the surgery by defining so-called "no-go" zones, areas that the surgeon wants to avoid (**Fig. 14**). Virtual geometrical regions within the 3D MR reconstructions can be defined, thereby outlining safe surgical corridors as well as anatomical structures to be avoided. When the surgeon encounters one of these defined boundaries, increasing force will be translated to the hand controller. In this manner, collisions can

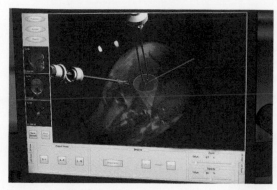

**Fig. 14.** With the neuroArm, virtual geometrical regions can be delineated within the 3D MR reconstructions using specially designed software. This means that safe surgical corridors as well as no-go zones—anatomical structures to be avoided—can be outlined. An increased force felt in the hand controllers signals the surgeon when one of these boundaries is encountered. This is an additional safety feature that the neurosurgeon can use during surgery. In this phantom experiment, the boundaries of the no-go zone are shown in blue. The virtual tool overlay has also been incorporated. The red, green, and blue lines define X,Y, and Z planes relative to the image and the centre of the safe surgical corridor.

be preempted and, together with such other software features as motion and force scaling, injury to normal brain tissue is minimized.

## Computer Applications

NeuroArm has four main software applications running concurrently on separate computers. The first is a command and status display, the main graphical control interface. It shows the 3D virtual scene of the manipulators and the surgical corridor in relation to the potential obstacles, such as the radio frequency (RF) coil and the magnet bore. The second is the MRI display, which provides 2D and 3D reconstructed images of the patient anatomy with optional tool overlay. The third application is the hand controller interface to the left and right haptic hand controllers. The last application is the controller interface to the manipulators and other required hardware. The software applications run on four computers because of the heavy workload, the demand for real-time response, and space limitations at the workstation. User Datagram Protocol/Internet Protocol messaging over gigabit Ethernet is used as the communication mechanism between the different elements of the software system.

Several mechanisms are in place to prevent unintended actions of the robot, a significant safety concern. Safety-critical software actions, such as turning on power or enabling manipulator motion, always require additional hardware action as confirmation. The concept of *state machines* has been incorporated into the software so that transition from one state to another occurs under tight control, with the simultaneous assessments of the safety level. In addition, software applications can detect potential collisions between the robot and any obstacles within the surgical field.

### Stereotaxy and Microsurgery

During a stereotactic procedure, one of the manipulators is transferred from the mobile base to an extension board attached to the head of the operating room table (**Fig. 15**). MRIs are acquired intraoperatively to provide real-time information regarding tool position relative to the planned surgical corridor and the lesion. Robot movement is gated to image acquisition to prevent the RF impulses from corrupting the position data from the joint position sensors. The biopsy forceps or implantation device can be manipulated using a linear drive mechanism that provides accurate lesion targeting. Two MR-compatible cameras attached to the extension board of the operating table provide visualization of the patient, the manipulator, and tool position.

Image-guided microsurgery is performed outside the magnet bore. After the perioperative imaging has been acquired and the magnet has

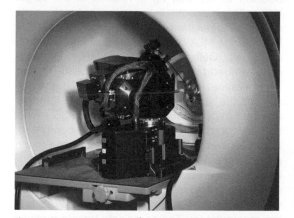

**Fig. 15.** NeuroArm setup for stereotaxy. Either of the manipulators can be transferred from the mobile base to an extension board attached to the head of the operating room table for stereotactic procedures. Two MR-compatible video cameras are also attached to the extension board to provide views of the patient, the manipulator, and the tool position. Real-time information of the tool position relative to the target lesion is acquired through intraoperative MR imaging, where the robot movement is gated to the image acquisition to minimize corruption of the position sensor data.

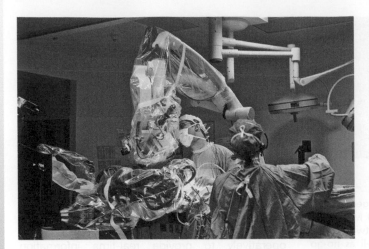

**Fig. 16.** NeuroArm in position during microsurgery. During surgery, the neuro-Arm is positioned next to the operating table, in place of the primary neurosurgeon. The positions of the microscope, the assistant, and the scrub nurse remain unchanged.

been retracted into its holding position, the robot can then be brought into position and registered to the images using the digitizing arm and RF coil fiducials. The manipulators may then be positioned in the place of the primary or assistant surgeon. The location of all other operating room personnel and standard equipment remains unchanged (**Fig. 16**). Even though microsurgery is performed outside the magnet bore, intraoperative imaging can be performed at any time during the surgery. To maintain image-guidance capability, reregistration is required each time neuroArm is brought back into the surgical field.

Registration allows the computer to know the position of the tool tip in relation to the target lesion. This is accomplished using the touch points on the manipulators and the RF coil, a six-DOF Microscribe MLX digitizing arm (Solution Technologies, Inc., Oella, Maryland), and MR-visible fiducials embedded in the RF coil head holder. Preoperative imaging is acquired with the RF coil. At the workstation, the MR-visible fiducials are then matched to those in a RF coil 3D model and the coordinate transformations are computed. At the operating table, coordinates of the touch points on the RF coil head holder and the manipulators are then acquired using the digitizing arm (**Fig. 17**). The touch-point data are then merged with a 3D model of the RF coil head holder and the manipulators. The coordinate transformations are again computed to complete the spatial registration of the robot to the MR image. Initial clinical experience using neuroArm has shown registration accuracy within 4 mm.

## Applications

After undergoing cadaveric and animal studies, neuroArm has been used in the surgical resection of tumor in five patients. Introduced in a gradual

manner, neuroArm has performed such tasks as thermocoagulation, microdissection, suction, and tissue removal, which would normally be performed by the primary neurosurgeon. The intraoperative MRI operating room has been converted from a 1.5-T to a 3-T platform. Modifications to neuroArm have been made to adapt to the higher magnetic field strength and change from local to room RF shielding. Through ongoing use, clinicians are gaining additional experience with the neuroArm.

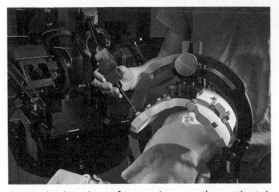

**Fig. 17.** Registration of neuroArm to the patient is necessary so that the computer can know the position of the tool tip in relation to the target lesion. After preoperative imaging is acquired with the RF coil head holder, the MR-visible fiducials within the coil are matched to those in a 3D model of the coil and coordinate transformations are computed at the workstation. At the operating table, coordinates of the touch points on the RF coil head holder and the manipulators are then acquired using neuroArm's six-DOF Microscribe MLX digitizing arm, seen here in a phantom study. The touch-point data are then merged with a 3D model of the RF coil head holder and the manipulators. The coordinate transformations are again computed to complete the spatial registration of the robot to the MR image.

## SUMMARY

Neurosurgical robots have the potential to push the limits of human technical capabilities. With the development of better imaging modalities and localization systems, the neurosurgical robot, with its enhanced ability for tool manipulation, can help neurosurgeons achieve greater precision and accuracy in accessing lesions through narrower surgical corridors. The ideal neurosurgical robot should blend accuracy, precision, reliability, and tireless consistency of the machine with human reasoning and adaptability. That ideal is nearly within our grasp.

## REFERENCES

1. Yasargil MG. A legacy of microneurosurgery: memoirs, lessons, and axioms. Neurosurgery 1999; 45(5):1025–92.
2. Hounsfield GN. Computerized transverse axial scanning (tomography): part I. Description of system. 1973. Br J Radiol 1995;68(815):H166–72.
3. Cormack AM. Reconstruction of densities from their projections, with applications in radiological physics. Phys Med Biol 1973;18(2):195–207.
4. Lauterbur PC. Progress in N.M.R. zeugmatography imaging. Philos Trans R Soc Lond B Biol Sci 1980; 289(1037):483–7.
5. Mansfield P, Maudsley AA. Medical imaging by NMR. Br J Radiol 1977;50(591):188–94.
6. Lunsford LD, Parrish R, Albright L. Intraoperative imaging with a therapeutic computed tomographic scanner. Neurosurgery 1984;15(4):559–61.
7. Black PM, Moriarty T, Alexander E III, et al. Development and implementation of intraoperative magnetic resonance imaging and its neurosurgical applications. Neurosurgery 1997;41(4):831–45.
8. Sutherland GR, Kaibara T, Louw D, et al. A mobile high-field magnetic resonance system for neurosurgery. J Neurosurg 1999;91(5):804–13.
9. Hall WA, Martin AJ, Liu H, et al. Brain biopsy using high-field strength interventional magnetic resonance imaging. Neurosurgery 1999;44(4):807–13.
10. Hadani M, Spiegelman R, Feldman Z, et al. Novel, compact, intraoperative magnetic resonance imaging–guided system for conventional neurosurgical operating rooms. Neurosurgery 2001;48(4): 799–807.
11. Kwoh YS, Hou J, Jonckheere EA, et al. A robot with improved absolute positioning accuracy for CT guided stereotactic brain surgery. IEEE Trans Biomed Eng 1988;35(2):153–60.
12. Drake JM, Joy M, Goldenberg A, et al. Computer and robot assisted resection of thalamic astrocytomas in children. Neurosurgery 1991;29(1):27–33.
13. Li QH, Zamorano L, Pandya A, et al. The application accuracy of the NeuroMate robot—a quantitative comparison with frameless and frame-based surgical localization systems. Comput Aided Surg 2002;7(2):90–8.
14. Varma TRK, Eldridge P. Use of the NeuroMate stereotactic robot in a frameless mode for functional neurosurgery. Int J Med Robot 2006;2(2):107–13.
15. Zimmermann M, Krishnan R, Raabe A, et al. Robot-assisted navigated neuroendoscopy. Neurosurgery 2002;51(6):1446–52.
16. Nimsky Ch, Rachinger J, Iro H, et al. Adaptation of a hexapod-based robotic system for extended endoscope-assisted transsphenoidal skull base surgery. Minim Invasive Neurosurg 2004;47(1):41–6.
17. Fankhauser H, Glauser D, Flury P, et al. Robot for CT-guided stereotactic neurosurgery. Stereotact Funct Neurosurg 1994;63(1–4):93–8.
18. Glauser D, Fankhauser H, Epitaux M, et al. Neurosurgical robot Minerva: first results and current developments. Comput Aided Surg 1995;1(5):266–72.
19. Chinzei K, Miller K. Towards MRI guided surgical manipulator. Med Sci Monit 2001;7(1):153–63.
20. Masamune K, Kobayashi E, Masutani Y, et al. Development of an MRI-compatible needle insertion manipulator for stereotactic neurosurgery. J Image Guid Surg 1995;1(4):242–8.
21. Le Roux PD, Das H, Esquenazi S, et al. Robot-assisted microsurgery: a feasibility study in the rat. Neurosurgery 2001;48(3):584–9.
22. Taylor RH, Jensen P, Whitcomb L, et al. A steady-hand robotic system for microsurgical augmentation. Int J Robot Res 1999;18(12):1201–10.
23. Fleming I, Balicki M, Koo J, et al. Cooperative robot assistant for retinal microsurgery. Med Image Comput Comput Assist Interv Int Conf Med Image Comput Comput Assist Interv 2008;11(Pt 2):543–50.
24. Hongo K, Kobayashi S, Kakizawa Y, et al. NeuRobot: telecontrolled micromanipulator system for minimally invasive microneurosurgery—preliminary results. Neurosurgery 2002;51(4):985–8.
25. Goto T, Hongo K, Kakizawa Y, et al. Clinical application of robotic telemanipualtion system in neurosurgery. Case report. J Neurosurg 2003;99(6):1082–4.
26. Hongo K, Goto T, Miyahara T, et al. Telecontrolled micromanipulator system (NeuRobot) for minimally invasive neurosurgery. Acta Neurochir Suppl 2006;98:63–6.
27. Gassert R, Burdet E, Chinzei K. Opportunities and challenges in MR-compatible robotics. IEEE Eng Med Biol Mag 2008;27(3):15–22.
28. Sutherland GR, Kelly JJP, Boehm DW, et al. Ceramic aneurysm clips for improved MR visualization. Neurosurgery 2008;62(5):ONS400–6.
29. Greer AD, Newhook P, Sutherland GR. Human-machine interface for robotic surgery and stereotaxy. IEEE/ASME Transactions on MRI Compatible Mechatronic Systems 2008;13(3):355–61.

30. Sutherland GR, Latour I, Greer AD, et al. An image-guided magnetic resonance compatible surgical robot. Neurosurgery 2008;62(2):286–93.

31. Louw DF, Fielding T, McBeth PB, et al. Surgical robotics: a review and neurosurgical prototype development. Neurosurgery 2004;54(3):525–37.

32. Sutherland GR, Latour I, Greer AD. Integrating an image-guided robot with MRI. IEEE Eng Med Biol Mag 2008;27(3):59–65.

33. Riviere CN, Rader RS, Thakor NV. Adaptive canceling of physiological tremor for improved precision in microsurgery. IEEE Trans Biomed Eng 1998;45(7):839–46.

34. Ang WT, Pradeep PK, Riviere CN. Active tremor compensation in microsurgery. Engineering in Medicine and Biology Society 2004. IEMBS '04. 26th Annual International Conference of the IEEE; San Francisco, CA: September 1–5, 2004;1:2738–41.

# Implantation of Deep Brain Stimulator Electrodes Using Interventional MRI

Philip A. Starr, MD, PhD[a],*, Alastair J. Martin, PhD[c],
Paul S. Larson, MD[b]

## KEYWORDS

- Deep brain stimulation • Interventional MRI
- Surgical methods • Neurosurgery
- Subthalamic nucleus • Parkinson disease

In this article we describe our technical approach to interventional MRI (iMRI)–guided deep brain stimulator (DBS) placement. This description is based on 53 DBS lead insertions into the subthalamic nucleus (STN) in patients with Parkinson disease. The conceptual foundation for the iMRI approach to STN-DBS derives from prior experience of our group and that of others with the standard technique: frame-based stereotaxy with microelectrode guidance. The criteria for successful STN lead placement have been physiologic (region in which microelectrode recording detected STN cells, including cells with movement-related responses) or clinical (lead placements that resulted in successful reduction in parkinsonian symptoms). During the past 10 years, many groups have, on a post hoc basis, correlated lead location by postoperative MRI with single-unit physiology,[1–4] thresholds for stimulation-induced adverse events,[5–7] and clinical success.[6,8–15] These papers have shown that the STN can be seen on MRI by its T2 hyperintensity,

and that the dorsolateral region of the MRI-defined STN reliably contains movement-related cells. Brain coordinates predicting clinical success have been elucidated.[6,8–15] This experience provided a conceptual justification for the use of imaging criteria alone to define and confirm accuracy of target placement.

## DESCRIPTION OF PROCEDURE

The technique evolved as an extension of the prior work of Hall and Truwit[16,17] in high-field iMRI-guided brain biopsy. The prior biopsy work used a smaller "joystick" aiming device (Medtronic Navigus) while the present work employed a skull-mounted device (Medtronic Nexframe) that has a "rotate/translate" mechanism, providing finer control at the expense of a less-intuitive aiming paradigm (**Fig. 1**).

Our approach uses a standard configuration (closed bore) 1.5-T MRI located in a radiology suite rather than an "intraoperative" MRI specifically

This work was supported by research grants from Medtronic Inc. (2004–2006) and Surgivision Inc. (2007–2008) to all three authors. Philip A. Starr and Paul S. Larson also received honoraria for speaking engagements from Medtronic Inc.

a Department of Neurosurgery, University of California, San Francisco, 533 Parnassus Avenue Box 0445, San Francisco, CA 94143, USA
b Department of Neurosurgery, University of California San Francisco, San Francisco, 505 Parnassus Avenue, Moffitt 779, San Francisco, CA 94143, USA
c Department of Radiology, University of California, San Francisco, 505 Parnassus Avenue, San Francisco, CA 94143, USA
* Corresponding author.
E-mail address: starrp@neurosurg.ucsf.edu (P.A. Starr).

Neurosurg Clin N Am 20 (2009) 207–217
doi:10.1016/j.nec.2009.04.010
1042-3680/09/$ – see front matter © 2009 Elsevier Inc. All rights reserved.

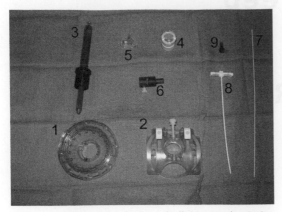

**Fig. 1.** Components of the skull-mounted aiming system (Nexframe and accessories). (1) Base of Nexframe. (2) Top of Nexframe. (3) Fluid-filled alignment stem. (4) Multilumen insert. (5) Bridge for multilumen insert. (6) Lead holder. (7) Ceramic stylet. (8) Peel-away sheath. (9) Depth stop for ceramic stylet.

configured for neurosurgery. This approach has five key features:

- Planning, insertion, and MRI confirmation of DBS lead placement are integrated into a single procedure while the patient is on the magnetic resonance (MR) gantry.
- The platform for inserting the DBS lead is a burr hole–mounted trajectory guide rather than a traditional stereotactic frame-and-arc system.
- Target coordinates are defined with respect to the MRI isocenter rather than with respect to a separate stereotactic space using fiducial markers.
- Patients are under general anesthesia in the supine position and no microelectrode recordings or test stimulation are performed.
- Target images are acquired after the burr hole is made and air enters the intracranial space, reducing the potential for errors associated with "brain shift," which can occur with conventional techniques in between image acquisition and probe insertion.

MR protocols used for each step are described in **Table 1**, and the key MR-compatible surgical instruments are shown in **Fig. 2**.

### Patient Preparation and Positioning

The patient is allowed to take his or her usual morning dose of antiparkinsonian medications. After premedication with midazolam and fentanyl, general anesthesia is induced with propofol in a room adjacent to the MRI suite. Anesthesia is maintained with sevoflurane and intermittent fentanyl and vecuronium boluses. Ventilation is adjusted to maintain end-tidal carbon dioxide between 35 and 40 mm Hg. After placement of an intra-arterial catheter into the wrist, the patient's head is placed into a carbon-fiber head holder designed to mount directly to the MRI gantry. The head holder is shown in **Fig. 3**. The frontal area is shaved using clippers. An array of four flexible surface coils positioned at the sides, top, back, and front of the head, is used for optimal MR signal acquisition.

### Trajectory Planning for Burr Hole Location

The patient is then moved into the bore of the MRI. An MRI-compatible anesthesia machine is used. The MR gantry is landmarked on the frontal scalp near the presumed coronal suture and advanced to magnet isocenter. A gadolinium-enhanced volumetric gradient echo MRI is obtained (scan parameters in **Table 1**, Protocol 1) parallel to the line between the anterior commissure and posterior commissure (AC-PC line). On the MR console, approximate anatomic targets are selected bilaterally at a point 12 mm lateral, 3 mm posterior, and 4 mm inferior to the midcommissural point. This preliminary target is used only for trajectory planning; final anatomic target selection is performed in a subsequent step described below. Single-slice obliqued parasagittal reformatted images are reconstructed and centered on the approximate targets; the surgeon can then view a variety of obliqued images all passing through the target to determine the trajectory options to the target. A trajectory that avoids sulci and cortical veins is then selected on the oblique image (**Fig. 4**). At the point where the trajectory crosses the scalp, a rapidly updating "MRI fluoroscopy" sequence (**Table 1**, Protocol 2, described below) is prescribed with its center at the intended entry. The surgeon reaches into the bore of the magnet and manually places an MR-visible pointer at the intended entry (**Fig. 5**A). The entry point is marked with a pen and the patient is moved to the back of the bore. Two nonsterile Nexframes are placed over the entry points to make sure there would be space between them (**Fig. 5**B), and the skull is marked percutaneously by injecting methylene blue through a 22-gauge needle at the scalp entry site (**Fig. 5**C).

### Initial Exposure and Mounting of Trajectory Guide

The frontal area is prepped and draped with an MRI bore drape designed to keep the surgical field sterile yet tolerate head movement between the center and back of the bore (a distance of ~1 m). A pressurized nitrogen tank and electrical power sources for bipolar cautery, one headlight, and one floor light are placed outside the MRI room with the regulator hose and electrical cords directed through a waveguide. Monopolar cautery is not used. After making coronally oriented incisions, 14-mm frontal burr holes are drilled with an MR-compatible cranial drill. The base rings for the Stimloc lead anchoring device and the Nexframe DBA ("deep brain access") trajectory guides are mounted over the burr holes. The dura mater is opened bilaterally and the leptomeninges is coagulated. The trajectory guide alignment stems are filled with sterile saline and mounted into the trajectory guide (**Fig. 6**A).

### Target Definition and Aiming of Alignment Stem

The patients is moved to reposition the head at magnet isocenter. Table movement is then disabled and no further patient movement is allowed until the leads are inserted and placement confirmed by imaging. A high-resolution T2 axial MRI is performed with 2-mm slice thickness, aligned such that one slice passes 4 mm inferior to the commissures (Protocol 3 in **Table 1**). The brain target is selected on this image (**Fig. 7**). The intended target is generally very close to the "default" coordinates of 12 mm lateral, 3 mm posterior, and 4 mm inferior to the midcommissural point. However, small adjustments in the default coordinates are made based on direct visualization of the borders of STN and red nucleus, so as to place the target within dorsolateral STN at least 2 mm from medial, lateral, and posterior borders. Axial and coronal volumetric T2 MRIs are acquired through the pivot points of the alignment stems (Protocol 4, **Table 1**). The pivot point is a sphere at the bottom of the alignment stem, which is situated at the center of rotation of the Nexframe and therefore remains fixed in space regardless of the Nexframe's orientation. The XYZ coordinates of target and pivot, with respect to MR isocenter, are determined by placing a "region of interest" cursor over the desired location. The final XYZ of the pivot is a synthesis of the values on coronal and sagittal views. These two points (target and pivot) define the "target line."

For the first side to be implanted, the XYZ coordinates of target and pivot are used to prescribe the "MR fluoroscopy" sequence (**Table 1**, Protocol 2). The scan is prescribed such that it is perpendicular to and centered on the target line at a location 9 to 10 cm superior to the burr hole.

The fluid stem is visible in this imaging volume. The surgeon dons a sterile hood to maintain the sterile field and reaches into the bore of the magnet to manually align the stem to the target line, while viewing the MR fluoroscopy image on an in-room monitor (see Video at www.neurosurgery.theclinics.com). When the desired alignment is achieved, the Nexframe is locked into place. Rapid, low-resolution oblique coronal and sagittal images (Protocol 5, **Table 1**) are obtained along the orientation of the stem, and the final anticipated target is reconstructed graphically (**Fig. 8**). Occasionally, the oblique scans predict a trajectory not perfectly aligned with the intended target. In these cases, a new alignment scan is prescribed with its center slightly modified and a new manual alignment is performed by the surgeon. The distance from the target to the relevant level of the trajectory guide (the step-off between thick and thin sections of the alignment stem) is measured on the oblique images to allow calculation of the position of the depth stop in the subsequent step. This distance is increased by 4.5 mm so that the peel-away sheath and stylet will slightly overshoot the target.

### Insertion of Guidance Sheath and Lead

The alignment stem is replaced with a five-channel multilumen insert, and a ceramic stylet within a plastic peel-away sheath is placed into the center lumen (**Fig. 6**B). A depth stop is placed on the stylet at the appropriate length as described above. The stylet/sheath assembly is advanced into the brain in two or three stepwise movements, monitored via in-plane MRI, using oblique sagittal and coronal T2 sequences (Protocol 6 in **Table 1**) (**Fig. 9**). The alignment and insertion procedure is then repeated for the contralateral side. A high-resolution axial T2 image is obtained through the target area to assess sheath/stylet position at the target (Protocol 3, **Table 1**) (**Fig. 10**).

If the placement of the peel-away sheath/stylet assembly is found to be inappropriate for either side (defined as distance between intended and actual stylet position of greater than 2 mm in the axial plane 4 mm below the commissures), a side channel of the Nexframe multilumen insert is considered to provide a parallel track with an offset of 3 mm in a direction perpendicular to the lead trajectory. If an offset of 3 mm does not provide an appropriate placement, the sheath/stylet is removed, the alignment stem is replaced, and the Nexframe trajectory is readjusted by repeating the alignment scans.

Two 28-cm DBS leads (Medtronic model 3389–28) are prepared by replacing their standard wire stylet with custom-made nonferrous titanium wire

**Table 1**
MRI pulse sequences for iMRI-guided DBS

| | Protocol Type and Purpose | | | | | | | |
|---|---|---|---|---|---|---|---|---|
| | Protocol 1. Volumetric Gadolinium-enhanced (T1 3D Gradient Echo) | Protocol 2. MR "Fluoroscopy" Sequence | Protocol 3. High-resolution Axial T2-weighted Fast Spin Echo (T2-FSE) | Protocol 4. Volumetric T2-weighted Fast Spin Echo (3D T2 FSE) | Protocol 5. Low-resolution T2-weighted Fast Spin Echo (T2-FSE) | Protocol 6. High-resolution T2-weighted Fast Spin Echo (T2-FSE) | Protocol 7. Intermediate-resolution T2-weighted Fast Spin Echo (T2-FSE) | Protocol 8. High-resolution Volumetric (T1 3D Gradient Echo) |
| Purpose | Trajectory planning | Marking of scalp entry point and aligning the fluid-filled stem | Identification of STN target point and confirmation of stylet position | Identification of the alignment stem pivot points | Confirmation of trajectory of alignment stem | Confirmation of trajectory of stylet during brain entry | Confirmation of lead depth | Measurement of postplacement lead location |
| Acquisition plane | Axial | Oblique axial | Axial | Coronal and sagittal | Oblique coronal and sagittal | Oblique coronal and sagittal | Axial | Axial |
| Slice thickness (mm) | 2.0 | 1.2 | 2.0 | 1.0 | 2.0 | 1.0 | 1.0 | 1.5 |
| Field of view (mm) | 260 × 207 | 128 × 104 | 260 × 222 | 256 × 256 | 250 × 188 | 256 × 216 | 256 × 192 | 260 × 222 |

| | | | | | | | | |
|---|---|---|---|---|---|---|---|---|
| Number of slices | 75 | 1 | 21 | 9 | 1 | 11 | 15 | 120 |
| Repetition time (mm) | 20 | 5.5 | 3000 | 2000 | 2000 | 2000 | 3000 | 20 |
| Echo time (mm) | 2.9 | 2.8 | 90 | 100 | 56 | 96 | 90 | 3.2 |
| Matrix size (mm) | 176 × 114 | 128 × 103 | 384 × 224 | 256 × 256 | 256 × 192 | 256 × 172 | 256 × 192 | 192 × 152 |
| Flip angle | 30° | 60° | 90° | 90° | 90° | 90° | 90° | 30° |
| Number of excitations | 1 | 1 | 6 | 1 | 2 | 1 | 1 | 1 |
| Echo train length | Not applicable | Not applicable | 16 | 54 | 24 | 56 | 42 | Not applicable |
| Bandwidth (kHz) | 54 | 75 | 40 | 182 | 115 | 160 | 88 | 50 |
| Specific absorption rate (W/kg) | 0.3 | 0.9 | 1.0 | 0.8 | 1.2 | 1 | 0.5 | 0.3 |
| Scan time (min:s) | 4:09 | 5 frames/s[a] | 8:42 | 1:28 | 0:18 | 1:22 | 4:06 | 8:54 |

[a] Each scan duration is 600 ms, but scans are "stacked" so as to present at 5 frames/s.

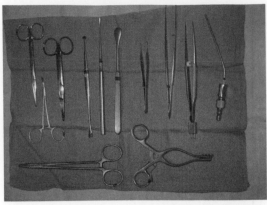

Fig. 2. MR-compatible titanium instruments for iMRI-guided DBS. (*Top row, left to right*) Metzenbaum scissors, hemostat, Mayo scissors, Penfield 1 and 2, Penfield 4, periosteal elevator, Adson toothed forceps, long toothed forceps, bipolar tips, #9 Fraser suction tip. (*Bottom row, left to right*) Needle holder, self-retaining retractor.

stylets supplied by Medtronic, Inc., so as to allow imaging of the lead with their wire stylets in place, without excessive artifact. On one side, the ceramic stylet is removed leaving the peel-away sheath in place and a "bridge" snapped over the multilumen insert. The bridge, which provides a space between itself and the multilumen insert for the sides of the peel-away sheath, contains a lead-holding screw. A depth stop is placed on the lead 42.5 mm higher than the depth stop on the ceramic stylet (to account for the extra height of the bridge and lead holder) and the lead is advanced through the sheath to target. Lead insertion is repeated on the contralateral side (**Fig. 6**C). An axial T2-weighted MRI is used to confirm lead depth (**Table 1**, Protocol 7).

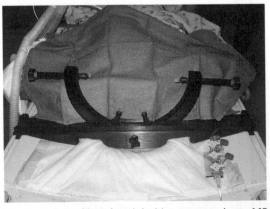

Fig. 3. Carbon fiber head holder mounted on MR gantry. A radio frequency receiving coil with a protective covering has been placed under the head holder.

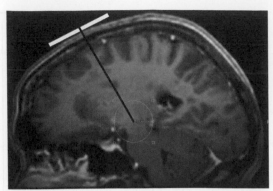

Fig. 4. Planning the entry point from an oblique refor-matted MR image passing through the target (**Table 1**, Protocol 1). The image plane was selected to pass through the target and to avoid the lateral ventricle. The black line represents the intended trajectory through the brain. The MR fluoroscopy sequence is prescribed at the surface of the scalp (*white line*), with its center at the intended entry point. The thin yellow circle is a "region of interest" marker centered on the approximate intended target.

## Closure, Final Imaging, and Implantable Pulse Generator Placement

The patient is moved to position the head at the back of the bore for easier surgical access. The peel-away sheaths are removed. The DBS leads are anchored to the skull with the Stimloc clips. The titanium wire stylets are removed from the leads, and the Stimloc cranial caps are set in place. The Nexframe trajectory guides are removed and the scalp is closed with sutures. The mean surgical time (from initial scalp incision to scalp closure) is 225 ± 30 minutes for simultaneous bilateral implants, and 217 ± 62 minutes for unilateral implantation.

The patient is moved back to isocenter for a final high-resolution volumetric T1-weighted MRI (**Table 1**, Protocol 8), this one for measuring lead-tip location and trajectory. The patient is awakened, recovers in the postanesthesia care unit, is monitored overnight in a step-down unit, and is discharged the day after lead implantation. Lead extenders and dual-channel pulse generator (Medtronic Kinetra) are placed 1 to 2 weeks later in the standard operating room.

## BRAIN PENETRATIONS USING THE INTERVENTIONAL MRI APPROACH

In 46 implants (87%) only a single brain penetration with the peel-away guidance sheath was necessary to place the lead at the final location. In 4 implants (8%), the first placement of the

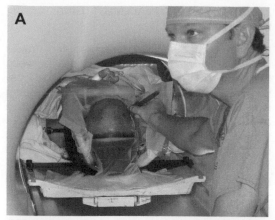

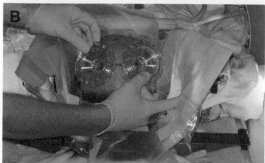

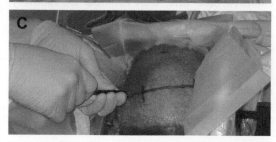

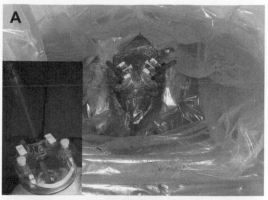

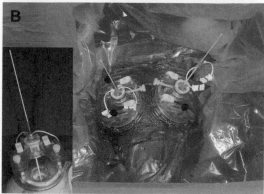

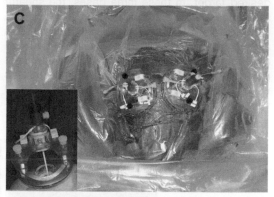

**Fig. 5.** Marking the entry point on the scalp surface. (*A*) The surgeon reaches into the magnet isocenter to place the tip of a nonsterile fluid-filled alignment stem at the center of the MR fluoroscopy sequence prescribed as shown in **Fig. 4**. The surgeon watches the in-room monitor for this step. The desired point is marked on the scalp with a pen. (*B*) After both intended entry sites are marked, the surgeon places two nonsterile Nexframe bases over the entries to make sure there is adequate space between them. (*C*) The surgeon makes a mark on the skull at the entry point by injecting a small amount of methylene blue under the scalp marking.

**Fig. 6.** Nexframe aiming device mounted on the skull at MR isocenter during various stages of the procedure. For each step, the insert at left shows a lateral view of the Nexframe (mounted on a model skull). (*A*) Alignment stems in place, immediately after the alignment to target. (*B*) Alignment stems have been replaced by the multilumen insert, with ceramic stylet and peel-away sheath inserted in the center channel. (*C*) After MR confirmation of the correct stylet position (see **Fig. 10**), the ceramic stylet is removed, and replaced with the bridge, lead holder, and 28-cm DBS lead.

stylet/sheath, at target depth, was considered inaccurate based on a greater than 2-mm radial error (measured in the plane 4 mm below the commissures). In these cases, the sheath/stylet was withdrawn completely and replaced either through a parallel port of the multilumen insert (three cases), or by replacing the alignment stem into the Nexframe and performing a new target

alignment (1 case). In another three implants, the sheath/stylet was advanced only partially into the brain on the first pass, and removed because the projected sheath/stylet trajectory, based on

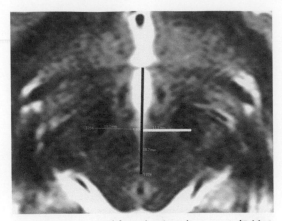

**Fig. 7.** MR image used for selecting the target. (**Table 1**, Protocol 3). This axial image is 4 mm below the AC-PC line. The black line is the projection of the AC-PC line onto this plane. The thick white line points from midline to the left STN target, in this case a distance of 11.2 mm. The thin white line is an annotation made with the MR software pointing to the right STN target.

oblique sagittal and coronal images in the plane of the sheath/stylet, appeared to predict a greater than 2-mm distance between intended and desired target. In these three cases, the sheath/stylet was removed, the alignment stem replaced, a new target alignment was performed with the alignment stem, and the sheath/stylet advanced a second time. The total number of instrument passes into the brain for the 53 DBS lead implants was 60. The maximum number of passes per lead was three.

## ACCURACY OF LEAD PLACEMENT USING INTERVENTIONAL MRI

In each procedure, we measured the "radial error," defined as the scalar distance between the location of the intended target and actual location of the ceramic stylet, in the axial plane 4 mm inferior to the commissures, on high-resolution axial T2 images. The mean ($\pm$ SD) radial error for the initial pass of the peel-away sheath/ceramic stylet assembly was 1.18 $\pm$ 0.65 mm. (The mean "final-pass" radial error was lower than the first-pass radial error because, in some cases, a second or third pass was made based on excessive first-pass distance between intended and actual stylet position.)

## COMPLICATIONS

There were no MRI-visible hemorrhages (either symptomatic or asymptomatic) in the 53 STN implantations. Two hardware infections occurred early in the series, both at the frontal incision (implants #7 and #11), requiring removal of all implanted hardware. One of these was accompanied by cerebritis, requiring a prolonged stay in the intensive care unit, with eventual full recovery. Both of these occurred before the availability of an MRI-compatible cranial drill. At that time, the parts of the procedure involving initial exposure and creation of the burr hole had to be performed in the room adjacent to the MRI room. Then the patient was moved into the MRI bore with partial re-draping of the field (described in reference[18]). Since the introduction of an MRI-compatible drill

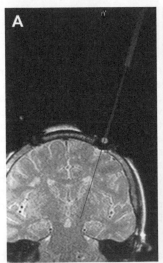
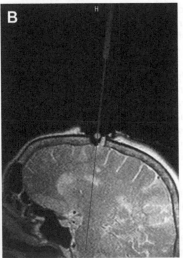

**Fig. 8.** Oblique coronal (*A*) and sagittal (*B*) MR images (**Table 1**, Protocol 5), taken after the alignment step shown in the Video. The images are taken in the plane of the intended trajectory. The dotted red line is an annotation on the MR monitor that shows the alignment stem trajectory, projected through the STN target.

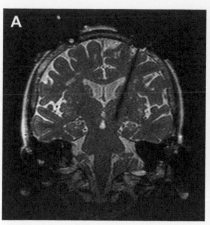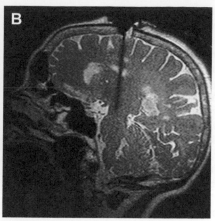

**Fig. 9.** Oblique coronal (*A*) and sagittal (*B*) MR images (**Table 1**, Protocol 6), same planes as **Fig. 8**, taken after advancing the ceramic stylet and peel-away sheath through the multilumen insert to the target.

and performance of all parts of the implant in the MRI room with a single draping procedure (beginning with implant #12), no further infections associated with the iMRI procedure have occurred.

In one patient, both leads were found to be inadequately placed, based on failure to achieve expected clinical results following multiple programming attempts. In retrospect, this patient had unusual STN anatomy (medially located STNs), a variant that was not fully appreciated on the targeting MRI, such that the intended target in the iMRI procedure did not reflect actual STN position. Expected clinical benefit was achieved following surgical replacement of the lead to a more medial location (10 mm from the midline), using the traditional stereotactic method.

In a historical comparison group of 76 STN-DBS electrodes implanted using traditional frame-based stereotaxy and routine postoperative MRI,[6] there were two hemorrhages (one symptomatic and one asymptomatic), no hardware infections, and one suboptimally placed lead that required surgical repositioning.

## FUTURE DEVELOPMENT OF INTERVENTIONAL MRI–GUIDED DEEP BRAIN STIMULATOR PLACEMENT

A long-range goal is to streamline the iMRI approach to DBS implantation so that it can be performed quickly within any diagnostic MRI scanner and without special modification for surgery. The iMRI approach in its current form has several cumbersome aspects:

Reaching into the bore of the magnet for manual steering is awkward, especially for those with short reach. This could be addressed with a mechanical remote control.

There is some loss of image quality with surface coils compared with rigid "birdcage" coils.

Because the availability of side channels is limited and because materials used to manufacture the multilumen insert make it impossible to interpolate smaller distances between center and side channels, the

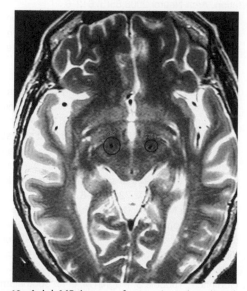

**Fig. 10.** Axial MR image of ceramic stylets (inside of peel-away sheath) at target. The intended targets are in the centers of the black circles. One stylet is within 0.5 mm of the intended target on the right. The other stylet is 1.2 mm posteromedial to the intended target on the left. These positions were considered adequate to proceed with lead implantation.

current trajectory guide is not optimized to deal with targeting errors.

The MR console does not have easy turnkey software to perform this procedure, and requires an operator with detailed technical knowledge of the software provided by the MR manufacturer. Moreover, the accuracy of many steps in the procedure relies on the operator's ability to accurately identify the geometric center of the pivot point and fluid stem.

The technique now requires in-room visualization by the surgeon of the MR "fluoroscopy" images used to manually perform the stem alignment. Expensive manufacturer-installed in-room monitors could be replaced by a simpler monitor projector set-up, as has been described for MRI-guided cardiac interventions.[19]

## SUMMARY

For the placement of DBSs, we have developed a technical approach that adapts the procedure to a standard-configuration 1.5-T diagnostic MRI scanner in a radiology suite. The technique uses near real-time MRI, in conjunction with a skull-mounted aiming device, as the sole method of guiding DBS electrodes to the STN and confirming localization. This technique may lead to more rapid lead implantation with greater patient comfort than is possible using standard physiologically guided techniques.

## ACKNOWLEDGMENTS

We thank Lynn Otten of Medtronic Inc. for providing custom-made titanium wire stylets for the Medtronic model 3389–28 DBS lead. We thank Elaine Lanier, Robin Taylor, and Jamie Grace for administrative assistance with preparation of the annual submission of the research protocol to the Institutional Review Board.

## APPENDIX: SUPPLEMENTARY MATERIAL

Supplementary material can be found, in the online version, at doi:10.1016/j.nec.2009.04.010

## REFERENCES

1. Abosch A, Hutchison WD, Saint-Cyr JA, et al. Movement-related neurons of the subthalamic nucleus in patients with Parkinson disease. J Neurosurg 2002; 97:1167–72.

2. Theodosopoulos PV, Marks WJ, Christine C, et al. The locations of movement-related cells in the human parkinsonian subthalamic nucleus. Mov Disord 2003;18:791–8.

3. Rodriguez-Oroz MC, Rodriguez M, Guridi J, et al. The subthalamic nucleus in Parkinson's disease: somatotopic organization and physiological characteristics. Brain 2001;124:1777–90.

4. Romanelli P, Heit G, Hill BC, et al. Microelectrode recording revealing a somatotopic body map in the subthalamic nucleus in humans with Parkinson disease. J Neurosurg 2004;100(4):611–8.

5. Ashby P, Kim YJ, Kumar R, et al. Neurophysiological effects of stimulation through electrodes in the human subthalamic nucleus. Brain 1999;122:1919–31.

6. Starr PA, Christine C, Theodosopoulos PV, et al. Implantation of deep brain stimulator electrodes into the subthalamic nucleus: technical approach and magnetic resonance imaging–verified electrode locations. J Neurosurg 2002;97:370–87.

7. Shields DC, Gorgulho A, Behnke E, et al. Contralateral conjugate eye deviation during deep brain stimulation of the subthalamic nucleus. J Neurosurg 2007;107(1):37–42.

8. Okun MS, Tagliati M, Pourfar M, et al. Management of referred deep brain stimulation failures: a retrospective analysis from 2 movement disorders centers. Arch Neurol 2005;62(8):1250–5.

9. Anheim M, Batir A, Fraix V, et al. Improvement in Parkinson disease by subthalamic nucleus stimulation based on electrode placement: effects of reimplantation. Arch Neurol 2008;65(5):612–6.

10. Plaha P, Ben-Shlomo Y, Patel NK, et al. Stimulation of the caudal zona incerta is superior to stimulation of the subthalamic nucleus in improving contralateral parkinsonism. Brain 2006;129(Pt 7):1732–47.

11. Saint-Cyr JA, Hoque T, Pereira LCM, et al. Localization of clinically effective stimulating electrodes in the human subthalamic nucleus on magnetic resonance imaging. J Neurosurg 2002;97:1152–66.

12. Lanotte MM, Rizzone M, Bergamasco B, et al. Deep brain stimulation of the subthalamic nucleus: anatomical, neurophysiological, and outcome correlations with the effects of stimulation. J Neurol Neurosurg Psychiatr 2002;72(1):53–8.

13. Zonenshayn M, Sterio D, Kelly PJ, et al. Location of the active contact within the subthalamic nucleus (STN) in the treatment of idiopathic Parkinson's disease. Surg Neurol 2004;62(3):216–25 [discussion: 225–16].

14. Godinho F, Thobois S, Magnin M, et al. Subthalamic nucleus stimulation in Parkinson's disease: anatomical and electrophysiological localization of active contacts. J Neurol 2006;253(10):1347–55.

15. McClelland S III, Ford B, Senatus PB, et al. Subthalamic stimulation for Parkinson disease: determination of electrode location necessary for clinical efficacy. Neurosurg Focus 2005;19(5):E12.

16. Hall WA, Liu H, Martin AJ, et al. Brain biopsy sampling by using prospective stereotaxis and a trajectory guide. J Neurosurg 2001;94:67–71.

17. Hall WA, Martin AJ, Liu H, et al. Brain biopsy using high-field strength interventional magnetic resonance imaging. Neurosurgery 1999;44:807–14.

18. Martin A, Larson P, Ostrem J, et al. Placement of deep brain stimulator electrodes using real-time high field interventional MRI. Magn Reson Med 2005;54:1107–14.

19. Guttman MA, Ozturk C, Raval AN, et al. Interventional cardiovascular procedures guided by real-time MR imaging: an interactive interface using multiple slices, adaptive projection modes and live 3D renderings. J Magn Reson Imaging 2007;26(6):1429–35.

# Future Applications: Gene Therapy

R.M. Richardson, MD, PhD*, V. Varenika, BS, J.R. Forsayeth, PhD,
K.S. Bankiewicz, MD, PhD

**KEYWORDS**

- Gene therapy • Convection enhanced delivery
- Restorative neurosurgery

Gene therapy for brain disorders is one of the most promising frontiers in the practice of restorative neurosurgery. There are significant experimental gene therapy initiatives underway that have led to currently active clinical trials using direct intracerebral delivery of viral vectors, and these treatments have been reported as safe and well tolerated. These studies include putaminal delivery of human aromatic L-amino acid decarboxylase (hAADC),[1] putaminal delivery of the neurotrophin neurturin,[2] and glutamic acid decarboxylase gene transfer to the subthalamic nucleus for Parkinson disease.[3] In the future, other clinical trials will likely use viral vectors to transfer genes that bestow on recipient tissue a desired enzymatic or neurotrophic activity relevant to the treatment of other neurodegenerative diseases, stroke, and traumatic brain injury.

The blood–brain barrier prevents significant amounts of most systemically administered agents from reaching therapeutic parenchymal levels without producing systemic toxicity. Although traditional direct local delivery of therapeutic agents into the brain relies on diffusion, resulting in nonhomogeneous distribution restricted to a few millimeters from the source, convection-enhanced delivery (CED) uses a pressure gradient established at the tip of an infusion catheter to distribute the therapeutic agent by bulk flow. This method produces an even distribution of highly concentrated agent over considerable distances, the volume of which depends on the structural properties of the tissue and the parameters of the infusion procedure.

Over the past decade, this laboratory has spearheaded nonclinical work in developing direct parenchymal CED of viral vectors for treating Parkinson disease. Multiple studies have demonstrated the efficacy of CED for distributing adeno-associated virus serotype 2 (AAV2) to specified brain regions, and an infusion cannula was designed to prevent vector infused under pressure from refluxing around the cannula. More recently, we have investigated the use of intraoperative MRI (iMRI) to guide infusions in real time, which provides the neurosurgeon with rapid feedback on the physical and anatomic diffusion parameters important for optimizing gene transfer and reducing the potential for adverse effects.

## IN VIVO GENE THERAPY: ADENO-ASSOCIATED VIRUS SEROTYPE 2 VECTORS

There are two broad categories of gene therapy: the direct transfer of a gene into the patient's own cells (in vivo), or the transplantation of cells genetically modified to perform a specific function (ex vivo). Clinical trials for Parkinson disease have used in vivo approaches, and these have shared in common the type of vector used for gene transfer: recombinant vectors derived from human adeno-associated virus serotype 2 (hAAV2). These vectors have been the most attractive of the candidate vector systems for gene transfer into neurons, because of the lack of any human disease associated with wild-type virus and the ability of AAV to transduce both dividing and nondividing cells.[4] Additionally, a consistently

Laboratory for Molecular Therapeutics, Department of Neurological Surgery, University of California San Francisco, 1855 Folsom Street, Room 226, San Francisco, CA 94103, USA
* Corresponding author.
E-mail address: richardsonma@neurosurg.ucsf.edu (R. Richardson).

Neurosurg Clin N Am 20 (2009) 219–224
doi:10.1016/j.nec.2009.04.004
1042-3680/09/$ – see front matter © 2009 Elsevier Inc. All rights reserved.

observed property of AAV2 is the extensive trafficking of vector from the site of infusion to distal anatomic locations, such as rapid transport of vector to globus pallidus after putaminal infusion.

Two key factors affect AAV2 trafficking, particularly relevant to iMRI imaging: the vasculature and axonal projections. CED studies in recipient rodents with and without a heartbeat demonstrated that cerebral fluid circulation through the perivascular space, powered by cardiac contractions, is the primary mechanism by which AAV2 and liposomes are spread within the brain.[5] Axonal distribution may occur through anterograde or retrograde transport, or by way of the periaxonal space in a manner similar to perivascular transport.[6] Additionally, distribution of infusate increases more rapidly in white matter, such as the corona radiata, than in the putamen and other gray matter.[7] Monitoring and control of viral vector trafficking thus presents a complex clinical challenge.

In our laboratory, extensive preclinical work in primates demonstrated that hAADC function, the generation of dopamine from L-dopa, is restored in the striatum following AAV2-hAADC delivery. AAV2-hAADC–treated monkeys showed increased responsiveness to L-dopa, as measured by positron emission tomography (PET), histology, and dopamine levels.[8] This work provided proof of principle for initiating clinical trials to deliver the hAADC gene to the human striatum in patients who have moderately advanced Parkinson disease. In a clinical trial involving our institution (NCT00229736), CED was used to infuse the post-commissural putamen bilaterally. In the first 5 patients treated in the lowest-dose cohort, PET imaging 6 months after the procedure showed a mean 30% increase in AADC activity.[1] Although postoperative T2-MRI and PET data obtained from 10 patients in the phase I AAV2-hAADC trial showed good overlap between the volume of distribution suggested by T2-MRI and the increase in PET signal, the overall infusion coverage of the putamen was variable from patient to patient.[9] In the absence of real-time visualization by iMRI, however, the extent to which this variation reflects actual target coverage cannot be determined.

## REAL TIME INTRAOPERATIVE MRI–BASED IMAGING OF CONVECTION-ENHANCED DELIVERY

The multifactorial nature of AAV2 trafficking alone suggests the need for real-time assessment of vector distribution. When the variables of the infusion procedure itself are also considered, however, real-time imaging becomes essential for optimizing clinical efficacy and safety. The goal is accurate delivery of therapeutic agents into target sites while minimizing exposure of untargeted tissue. Adequate visualization should confirm target coverage and detect reflux, leakage, anatomic deformation, and aberrant delivery. With these factors in mind, an iMRI-based method to visualize CED in real time was developed.

CED is an effective method for local delivery, not only of AAV but also of liposomes that are nanoscale carriers consisting of a phospholipid membrane shell surrounding a hollow core. Because liposomes can encapsulate a broad range of therapeutic agents and other small molecules, they were used to develop a real-time MR imaging method to track infused liposomes containing gadoteridol (GDL). MRI of liposomal GDL was found to be highly predictive in determining liposomal tissue distribution, as confirmed by histologic comparison with concomitant administration of fluorescent liposomes.[10]

Liposomal infusion studies demonstrate that differences in cytoarchitecture between structures infused, particularly between gray matter and white matter, are an anatomic determinant of infusate distribution. For instance, corona radiata infusions clearly show distribution following white matter fibers, whereas the limited size of the putamen restricts the allowable volume of infusion in that nucleus. In addition, the real-time liposomal infusion protocol has been used to identify important potential pitfalls for putaminal infusion. Anterior lateral leakage can be visualized by signal enhancement that follows the perivascular space of lateral striate arteries connecting to perivascular space of the medial cerebral artery, terminating in the Sylvian fissure and insular cortex.[11] Despite this potential for leakage, the real-time monitoring technique allows us to stop the infusion at any point, thereby permitting the filling of the putamen or similar structures with some precision.

An additional, related challenge is the leakage of infusate out of targeted parenchyma into adjacent sulci and ventricles. In a retrospective nonhuman primate study composed of 54 CED sessions monitored with real-time iMRI imaging, leakage occurred in approximately 20% of infusions.[12] Consequently, the distribution of liposomes within the target structure ceased to increase or was significantly attenuated after the onset of leakage. Escape of the agent from the targeted area, especially into the cerebrospinal fluid (CSF) space, potentially increases the risk for adverse and unexpected clinical events. This phenomenon may be reflected in mixed results reported from some clinical trials in which CED was used to infuse therapeutic agents in the absence of real-time visual guidance. For example, neutralizing antibodies have been reported in the CSF of some subjects after GDNF infusion into the putamen.[13,14]

Strategies for real-time iMRI-based imaging of AAV distribution during CED include coinfusion of nanoscale imaging agents or labeling of the viral capsid. Lonser's group[15] has demonstrated the coinfusion of radiolabeled AAV1 serotype capsids with ferumoxtran-10, a similarly sized (24 nm) super-paramagnetic iron oxide nanoparticle. This method was used to define clear hypointense regions of distribution visualized with real-time MRI, which were easily distinguishable from surrounding tissue in white and gray matter. The true volume of distribution of the viral capsid was confirmed by autoradiography, and the concentration of ferumoxtran-10 that most closely predicted AAV1 volume of distribution was determined. Similarly, recent studies in our laboratory have used coinfusion of GDL with AAV2 vector, whereby GDL distribution observed with real-time MRI corresponded well with the volume AAV2 transduction, as detected by

immunohistochemistry in the corona radiata (**Fig. 1**) and thalamus (**Fig. 2**). These efforts are the first to demonstrate real-time imaging of viral vector infusions in primate models, a critical step in bringing this technology into clinical practice.

Results from a double-blind, sham-controlled phase 2 trial of CERE-120 (AAV2-NTN), driving expression of human neurturin, a neurotrophic factor, were recently released.[16] This trial in 58 patients who had advanced Parkinson disease did not use CED for infusion of the viral vector and did not demonstrate an appreciable difference between patients treated with AAV2-NTN versus those in the control group. Careful analysis of these data will be required to ascertain whether a variable extent of target transduction, attributable to manual rather than convection-enhanced delivery, may have contributed to the negative results. Eventual use of iMRI-guided CED in all gene therapy clinical trials will be critical for separating issues related to agent delivery from those related to agent efficacy.

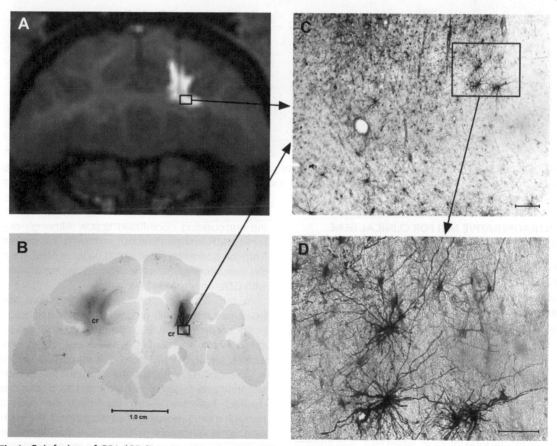

**Fig. 1.** Coinfusion of GDL (GD liposomes) and AAV1-GFP vector into the corona radiata. Successful distribution is demonstrated by MRI during vector administration (*A*) and 5 weeks post infusion using GFP-IR staining (*B*). GFP-expressing glia cells are well visualized at higher magnification (*C, D*).

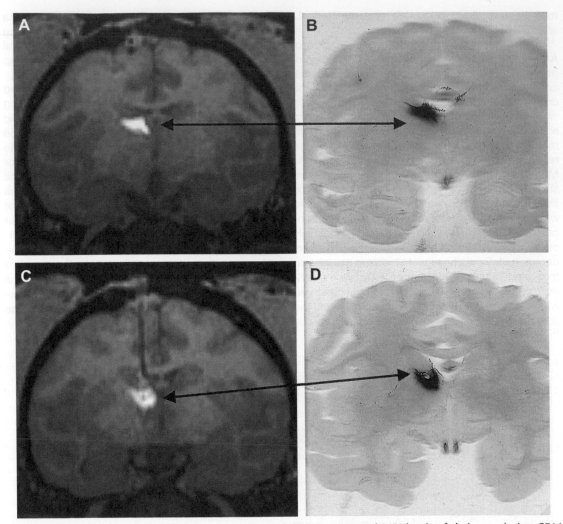

**Fig. 2.** Successful targeting of thalamus using GDL/AAV2-GFP. Two coronal MRI levels of thalamus during GDL/AAV-2-GFP administration (*A, C*) with corresponding histologic demonstration of neuronal GFP-expression in the thalamus (*B, D*).

## INTRAOPERATIVE MRI FOR CLINICAL GENE THERAPY

Real-time iMRI imaging of CED in the human brain has thus far not been used in gene therapy trials, although one case has been reported for the infusion of glucocerebrosidase into the frontal lobe and brainstem of a patient who had neuronopathic Gaucher disease.[17] A guide cannula was implanted for the procedure, the imaging and infusion were completed outside of the operating room, and the patient was returned to the operating room for cannula removal under a single session of general anesthesia. Although T2 and FLAIR sequences could not distinguish infusate distribution in the initial frontal lobe infusion, when GDL was coadministered for the brainstem infusion the infused anatomic region was clearly distinguished from the surrounding noninfused tissue. Although obtaining MR imaging without removing the patient from the operating room would be ideal, this report did validate the use of real-time imaging of CED with GDL coinfusion in humans.

At our institution, prospective stereotaxy has been used for iMRI-guided placement of deep brain stimulation (DBS) electrodes (see article elsewhere in this issue), wherein surgery is performed within the MR bore. The intubated patient is immobilized within the intraoperative MR scanner and imaging is performed to define the desired trajectory, with the electrode placed through a skull-mounted trajectory guide. We envision a modification of this technique for gene therapy, by adapting the CED infusion and cannula set-up used in the AAV2-hAADC clinical trial for use with the skull-mounted trajectory guide.

## CONTINUING TRANSLATIONAL RESEARCH

The refinement of nonclinical studies in nonhuman primates remains critical for driving subsequent CED gene therapy clinical trials that use iMRI. Primate studies have several advantages over rodent studies: greater anatomic, metabolic, and electrophysiologic similarity to the human brain; ability to model stereotactic and computer-assisted surgical techniques; ability to model parenchymal infusion characteristics, such as perivascular transport; analogous postoperative functional imaging; and ability for long-term (years) follow-up.[18] Primary problems that remain to be addressed in future studies include optimizing contrast agents for coinfusion with AAV vectors and verifying lack of neuronal damage with long-term follow-up, versus developing tagging methods for direct capsid labeling that do not alter vector function or receptor binding. As AAV infusion imaging improves, further studies will better elucidate mechanisms involved in leakage or spread of infusate from the intended target.

Additional disease paradigms should also be pursued. The structural anatomy that defines AAV trafficking in one disease may be altered in others. Eventual gene therapy strategies for neuroprotection, pertinent to treating stroke and traumatic brain injury, will have to overcome major macro- and microscopic structural alterations in brain tissue that will vary with injury mechanism, location, and acuity. Likewise, application of gene therapy to demyelinating diseases will have to consider the effect of demyelination on convection of the infusate through white matter tracts. Gene therapy targets, such as the subventricular zone and hippocampal dentate gyrus, areas of endogenous neurogenesis that harbor neural progenitor cells with the potential for therapeutic genetic reprogramming, offer a unique challenge because of the potential for vector leakage through neighboring ependyma and into the ventricular space.

## SUMMARY AND FUTURE CLINICAL APPLICATION

Gene therapy for Parkinson disease is progressing well as an experimental therapy because of an effective, safe vector system and a growing understanding of vector trafficking within the brain. The next major step forward is to translate experience with iMRI for DBS placement into protocols for real-time monitoring of the CED system for AAV2 infusion. Parkinson disease is the disease entity with which the field has entered the era of in vivo gene therapy, and efforts have initially been targeted toward alleviation of symptoms. Continued development of iMRI-CED will allow finer resolution of infused agent and better control of target coverage, which in turn will expand the potential clinical targets for in vivo gene therapy. Reliable visualization of viral infusate or surrogate, and subsequent ability to control the volume of distribution, will be absolute requirements for applying this technology in more severely damaged brain parenchyma, as occurs in stroke, traumatic brain injury, or demyelinating diseases.

## REFERENCES

1. Eberling JL, Jagust WJ, Christine CW, et al. Results from a phase I safety trial of hAADC gene therapy for Parkinson disease. Neurology 2008;70:1980.
2. Marks WJ Jr, Ostrem JL, Verhagen L, et al. Safety and tolerability of intraputaminal delivery of CERE-120 (adeno-associated virus serotype 2-neurturin) to patients with idiopathic Parkinson's disease: an open-label, phase I trial. Lancet Neurol 2008;7:400.
3. Kaplitt MG, Feigin A, Tang C, et al. Safety and tolerability of gene therapy with an adeno-associated virus (AAV) borne GAD gene for Parkinson's disease: an open label, phase I trial. Lancet 2007; 369:2097.
4. Hadaczek P, Kohutnicka M, Krauze MT, et al. Convection-enhanced delivery of adeno-associated virus type 2 (AAV2) into the striatum and transport of AAV2 within monkey brain. Hum Gene Ther 2006;17:291.
5. Hadaczek P, Yamashita Y, Mirek H, et al. The "perivascular pump" driven by arterial pulsation is a powerful mechanism for the distribution of therapeutic molecules within the brain. Mol Ther 2006; 14:69.
6. Varenika V, Dickinson P, Bringas J, et al. Detection of infusate leakage in the brain using real-time imaging of convection-enhanced delivery. J Neurosurg 2008 Nov;109(5):874–80.
7. Krauze MT, McKnight TR, Yamashita Y, et al. Real-time visualization and characterization of liposomal delivery into the monkey brain by magnetic resonance imaging. Brain Res Brain Res Protoc 2005; 16:20.
8. Bankiewicz KS, Forsayeth J, Eberling JL, et al. Long-term clinical improvement in MPTP-lesioned primates after gene therapy with AAV-hAADC. Mol Ther 2006;14:564.
9. Valles F, Eberling JL, Starr PA, et al. Imaging of AAV2-hAADC infusion in a Phase I study of AAV2-hAADC gene therapy for Parkinson's disease. NeuroImage, in press.
10. Saito R, Krauze MT, Bringas JR, et al. Gadolinium-loaded liposomes allow for real-time magnetic resonance imaging of convection-enhanced delivery in the primate brain. Exp Neurol 2005;196:381.

11. Krauze MT, Saito R, Noble C, et al. Effects of the perivascular space on convection-enhanced delivery of liposomes in primate putamen. Exp Neurol 2005;196:104.

12. Varenika V, Dickinson P, Bringas J, et al. Detection of infusate leakage in the brain using real-time imaging of convection-enhanced delivery. J Neurosurg 2008; 109:874.

13. Gill SS, Patel NK, Hotton GR, et al. Direct brain infusion of glial cell line-derived neurotrophic factor in Parkinson disease. Nat Med 2003;9:589.

14. Slevin JT, Gerhardt GA, Smith CD, et al. Improvement of bilateral motor functions in patients with Parkinson disease through the unilateral intraputaminal infusion of glial cell line-derived neurotrophic factor. J Neurosurg 2005;102:216.

15. Szerlip NJ, Walbridge S, Yang L, et al. Real-time imaging of convection-enhanced delivery of viruses and virus-sized particles. J Neurosurg 2007;107: 560.

16. Ceregene announces clinical data from phase 2 clinical trial of CERE-120 for Parkinson's disease. Available at: http://www.ceregene.com/press_112 608.asp. Accessed December 13, 2008.

17. Lonser RR, Schiffman R, Robison RA, et al. Image-guided, direct convective delivery of glucocerebrosidase for neuronopathic Gaucher disease. Neurology 2007;68:254.

18. Richardson RM, Larson PS, Bankiewicz KS. Gene and cell delivery to the degenerated striatum: status of preclinical efforts in primate models. Neurosurgery 2008;63:629.

# Future Directions: Use of Interventional MRI for Cell-Based Therapy of Parkinson Disease

Joshua Roskom[a], Andrzej Swistowski[b], Xianmin Zeng[c], Daniel A. Lim, MD, PhD[d,e],*

## KEYWORDS

- Embryonic stem cells • Induced pluripotent stem cells
- Cell transplantation • Parkinson's disease
- Dopamine neurons • Interventional MRI

Transplantation of neural cells for the treatment of neurologic disorders has garnered much attention and considerable enthusiasm from patients and physicians alike. Cell-based therapies have been proposed for a wide range of central nervous system pathologies ranging from stroke and trauma to demyelinating disorders and neurodegenerative diseases. Notably, cell transplantation for Parkinson disease (PD) has become even more attractive with the rapid advances in derivation of dopaminergic neurons from human embryonic stem cells (hESCs). The authors expect that grafting of hESC-derived dopaminergic neuronal progenitors will enter clinical testing in the next 4 to 5 years. To translate this cellular technology into an efficient surgical therapy, we will need to parallel the progress made on the cell biology front with advancements in neurosurgical approaches and devices for implantation of cells. Here, we briefly review some of the relevant issues regarding the transplantation of cells for treatment of PD and hypothesize how interventional MRI may be useful to optimize the surgical delivery of cells for PD and other central nervous system disorders.

## DOPAMINERGIC NEURON REPLACEMENT THERAPY FOR PARKINSON DISEASE

Although it is now recognized that neurodegeneration is widespread in PD, a pathologic characteristic of PD is the loss of the dopaminergic neurons that project axons from substantia nigra to a structure in the striatum called the putamen.[1] Because of the loss of these nigrostriatal neurons, the putamen is severely depleted of dopaminergic innervation,[2] and the degree of PD-related motor disability correlates with severity of this reduction.[3] Dopamine replacement in the form of the precursor levodopa has thus been the mainstay of PD treatment since the late 1960s[4] and provides dramatic benefit in early stages of the disease. Unfortunately, levodopa eventually becomes limited in its effectiveness with the development of motor complications, of which there are two primary forms. In one phenomenon, the patient becomes less responsive to levodopa therapy, with the effectiveness wearing off between doses, leaving the patient in an "off-time" state consisting of increased motor symptoms (akinesia, rigidity, resting tremor). The other

[a] Department of Neurological Surgery, University of California, San Francisco, 505 Parnassus Avenue, M779, Box 0112, San Francisco, CA 94143, USA

[b] Buck Institute for Age Research, 8001 Redwood Boulevard, Novato, CA 94945, USA

[c] North Bay California Institute for Regenerative Medicine (CIRM) Shared Research Laboratory for Stem Cells & Aging, Buck Institute for Age Research, 8001 Redwood Boulevard, Novato, CA 94945, USA

[d] Neurosurgical Section, Surgical Service, Department of Veterans Affairs, San Francisco Veterans Affairs Medical Center, 4150 Clement Street, San Francisco, CA 94121, USA

[e] Neurosurgical Section, Surgical Service, San Francisco Veterans Affairs Medical Center, Department of Veterans Affairs, 4150 Clement Street, Mail Stop 0112, San Francisco, CA 94121, USA

* Corresponding author.
E-mail address: limd@neurosurg.ucsf.edu (D.A. Lim).

Neurosurg Clin N Am 20 (2009) 225–232
doi:10.1016/j.nec.2009.04.005
1042-3680/09/$ – see front matter © 2009 Published by Elsevier Inc

form of motor complication is the development of levodopa-induced dyskinesias, which are abnormal, involuntary movements.[5,6] The causes of motor complications to levodopa therapy are not well understood. These limitations of levodopa therapy and the failure of other medical and surgical treatments to alter the progressive nature of PD have inspired investigations into restorative cell-based therapies.

Transplantation of dopaminergic cells for PD has the conceptual advantage of providing a continuous source of dopamine to the putamen and thus may ameliorate the aforementioned complications associated with chronic, intermittent levodopa therapy. Also, because some dopaminergic cells make synaptic connections with the host cells, transplants may provide a more physiologically relevant source of dopamine for neuronal activity.

### Early Trials Using Fetal Midbrain Tissue

The first successful transplantation of dopaminergic neuronal precursors to the putamen of patients with PD was performed in Sweden nearly 20 years ago.[7] These cells were obtained from the fetal midbrain of aborted embryos, and the grafted tissue harbored neuronal precursors that could integrate into the host,[8] produce dopamine,[9] and in some cases allow long-term reduction in levodopa dosage. Unfortunately, enthusiasm faded when double-blind trials revealed more marginal results (reviewed in Ref.[10]) as well as a side effect of graft-induced dyskinesias (GIDs) in 15% to 56% of the patients.[11,12] Furthermore, using fetal tissue as the source for clinical transplantation therapies has been deemed to be not practical because of a limited availability of donor tissue and because of ethical concerns.

### The Promise of Embryonic Stem Cells

In the early 1990s, investigators began asking if cultured stem cells could be used to produce dopaminergic neurons as an alternative to primary fetal tissue. Because stem cells can be greatly expanded in culture, large numbers of dopaminergic neurons could theoretically be produced as a routine (reviewed in Ref.[13]). In addition, transplantation of a more pure population of dopaminergic neurons (in comparison to the mixed neuronal population found in fetal graft tissue) might reduce the incidence of the GID side effect. Neural stem cells have been isolated and cultured from fetal and adult neural tissue; however, these cells have had limited potential to differentiate into dopaminergic neurons and produce therapeutic effect on transplantation (reviewed in

Ref.[14]). Given this present limitation, much attention has been directed to the use of embryonic stem cells (ESCs).

Mouse ESCs can be efficiently differentiated into dopaminergic neuronal precursors, and transplantation of these cells in a rodent model of PD restored function.[15] These studies were soon followed by those describing methods of differentiating human ESCs (hESCs) into precursors of dopaminergic neurons for transplantation.[16–28] It is now clear that authentic dopaminergic neurons can be generated from hESCs and that grafts can release dopamine and ameliorate behavioral deficits in rodent PD models. Here, we show an example of dopaminergic neurons derived from xeno- and serum-free adapted hESCs under good manufacturing practices–compliant conditions that are suitable for eventual human therapy (**Fig. 1**). These cells have confirmed midbrain dopaminergic neuron phenotypes by molecular expression analysis and neurochemical analysis. Transplantation of these cells results in behavioral recovery in a rat model of PD. There is now great excitement about the prospect of using hESC-derived precursors for transplantation therapy.

### Continued Advancements in Stem Cell Technologies: Autologous Stem Cells

One important concern regarding cell transplant therapies is the potential of immunorejection of the grafted cells (reviewed in Ref.[10]). To circumvent this potential problem, researchers have made progress in technologies to generate autologous stem cell populations, so that the induced dopaminergic cells are genetically and therefore immunologically identical to the recipient. Tabar and colleagues[29] recently derived mouse embryos by way of nuclear transfer using donor fibroblasts from mice with an experimental form of PD. These nuclear transfer ESCs (ntESCs) were differentiated into dopaminergic neurons and transplanted back into the donor mice. ntESC-derived dopaminergic neurons had improved survival and induced greater recovery, supporting the notion that immunologically matched cells may be of clinical benefit. Wernig and colleagues[30] took a different approach, using induced pluripotent stem cells (iPS cells) from mouse fibroblasts. iPS cells are generated from the enforced expression of four transcription factors in adult fibroblasts, and these cells behave similarly to ESCs, maintaining the ability to generate all differentiated cell types. Transplantation of dopaminergic cells derived from iPS cells also resulted in functional improvement in a rodent model of PD. Although there are logistical and potential safety problems with

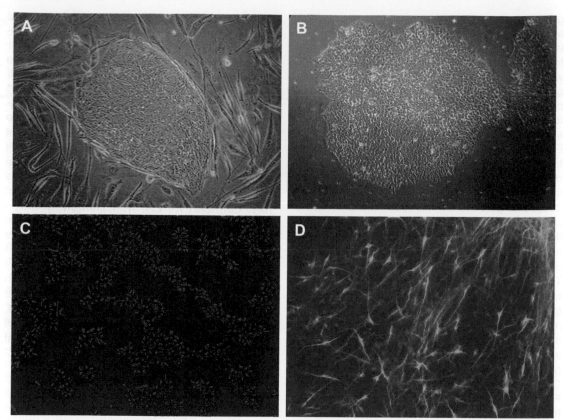

**Fig. 1.** Prolonged culture of hESCs in serum-free defined conditions differentiate into midbrain dopaminergic neurons efficiently. (*A*) Example of hESC colony on feeders monolayers. (*B*) hESC colony growing in serum-free defined medium. Neural induction of hESCs was initiated by fibroblast growth factor-2 by way of embryoid body formation. (*C*) A homogeneous population of Nestin+ neural precursors (*red*) was generated after 14 days of differentiation. (*D*) Neural precursors differentiated into dopaminergic neurons efficiently as evidenced by a high percentage of neurons stained positive for tyrosine hydroxylase (*green*) after 6 weeks of differentiation. Nuclei are counterstained by DAPI (*blue*).

producing such patient-specific cells for transplantation, it seems promising that such cells with low immmunorejection can be generated. iPS cells may not turn out to be the best source of cells for transplantation for PD: although most patients do not harbor known mutations for PD, there may be other genetic profiles that result in increased susceptibility to PD. Thus, while autologous cells from patients who have PD may have a lower immunorejection potential, there may be a greater risk for accelerated PD-like neurodegeneration in the grafted cells.

## Recent Studies of the Long-term Potential Viability of Cell Transplants for Parkinson Disease

Three recent reports have begun to address the question of long-term graft viability. In patients who received the fetal midbrain neural transplants, some of the surviving dopaminergic neurons exhibit pathologic changes associated with PD.[31,32] This finding has called into question the viability of the approach of cellular grafting for PD, because these case reports suggest that the diseased PD brain environment is toxic to the grafted neurons. In this case, it seems possible that any grafted cells could be threatened with disease process similar to PD. It should be noted, however, that only a few of the grafted neurons appeared to be affected, and another autopsy study of a transplanted patient who had PD did not reveal such pathologic changes.[33] Further studies are required to understand the durability of cell transplantation therapy for PD.

## POTENTIAL ADVANTAGES OF INTERVENTIONAL MRI FOR CELL TRANSPLANTATION
### Improved Accuracy of Graft Placement

One prerequisite for the success of cell transplantation therapy for PD is the accurate placement of grafts at the appropriate target locations. For transplantation of fetal dopaminergic cells in two large clinical trials involving patients who had PD, frame-based targeting with MRI-based stereotaxy was used. Although such stereotactic surgery based on internal brain landmarks (anterior and posterior commissures) with MRI guidance allows for targeting relatively small structures, such as the subthalamic nucleus, it is still prone to inaccuracy. For instance, in a nonhuman primate study of cell transplantation for PD, complete accuracy was only 80% (60 of 75 tracts) with nearly 7% of targets completely missed.[34] Some explanations for missed targets include the following: error in the precision of the frame, image distortion in an MRI field, brain shift due to loss or shift of cerebrospinal fluid (CSF) during surgery,[35] and displacement of brain under pressure of the advancing needle.[36] These inherent inaccuracies of indirect MRI-based targeting can be partially overcome by microelectrode recording[37–39]; however, such methods are relatively slow and require that the patient be awake for surgery. Because iMRI would allow for acquisition of targeting MRI after the entry burr hole is made, the problem of brain shift due to CSF leak and air entry is reduced considerably. Furthermore, after the cannula is placed at the intended target, another MRI can be immediately obtained so that the anatomic target is confirmed before cells are actually delivered into the brain. The prospective stereotaxis provided by iMRI thus greatly mitigates some of the limitations of indirect targeting. We anticipate that use of iMRI would provide the best and potentially safest method of cell delivery in a trial for PD.

Improved targeting and definition of target may reduce the likelihood of GIDs. Although it is not at all clear why GIDs appear in some patients, one notion is that this unwanted side effect results from patchy reinnervation of striatal regions resulting in unbalanced increases in dopaminergic function.[40] Theoretically, we would want to transplant only into the most dopamine-depleted regions as determined by[18] F-dopamine positron emission tomography (FD-PET) and do so in the most homogenous manner possible. Perhaps we will be able to fuse FD-PET images with MRI sequences obtained in the iMRI to improved definition of target, directing transplantation to the most dopamine-depleted areas of the putamen.

### Shortened Surgical Time

With continued advancements of the skull-mounted targeting device, MR interface and related software, and standardization of anesthesia delivery in the MR environment, we anticipate that the surgical time for intracranial stereotactic procedures will decrease substantially. This decrease is an inherent advantage for cell transplantation procedures; it is likely that cells prepared for implantation will have a limited "shelf life," with decreasing viability with increased preimplantation duration. By shortening the operative time, the time interval in which cells are in the relatively inhospitable environment of the cannula will be kept to a minimum.

## DEVELOPMENTS FOR INTERVENTIONAL MRI CELL TRANSPLANTATION
### New Cannulas for Cell Transplantation and Methods of Cell Tracking

Currently, iMRI is used for deep brain stimulation (DBS) implantation, and future developments in that technology are reviewed elsewhere in this issue. To bring iMRI to cell transplantation, modifications of the technique for DBS or gene therapy can be implemented, but one important consideration is the actual device used for the cell injection. The cannulas used in the Freed and colleagues[11,41] clinical trial and a more recent development[42] are both made of ferrous metals unsuitable for the high-field MR environment. We will thus need to use a cannula system made of titanium, ceramic, or plastics. The actual design of the cannula (eg, side port versus end port, or peel away) needs to be investigated.

It would also be ideal to have the dopaminergic cells labeled with an MR contrast agent to allow in vivo identification and tracking of the grafted cells. One particularly intriguing technology uses nanometer-sized iron oxide particles to label individual cells in vitro for later identification by MRI in vivo; such microscopic particles of iron oxide are superparamagnetic, resulting in a strong hypointensity on MR images (reviewed in Ref.[43]). Future developments in this technology may allow one to even more clearly distinguish live grafted cells from ones that have died.[44]

### Outline of a Proposed Interventional MRI Strategy for Transplantation of Human Embryonic Stem Cell–Derived Dopaminergic Neuronal Precursors

Here, we briefly outline general principles for a suggested surgical protocol for cell-based therapy of PD performed in an iMRI operative suite (**Fig. 2**). We assume here that motor regions of the putamen are the intended targets.

Preoperative acquisition of a high-resolution, volumetric MRI and an FD-PET scan. These images could be obtained up to several days before the operation.

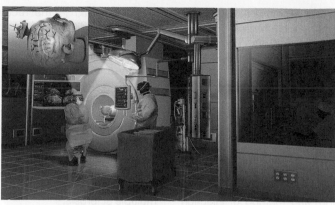

**Fig. 2.** Conceptual drawing of an iMRI suite used for cell transplantation, gene therapy, or DBS. At the left, the surgeon (seated) and scrub technician (standing) work together to first create the burr hole and attach the trajectory guide device. The inset at top left shows how the trajectory guide device is attached to the patient's skull to target the cannula to the desired intracranial location. The targeting and introduction of the cannula is a coordinated effort between the surgeon and another team member (shown here seated in the room at the right) who assists with image acquisition and MR fluoroscopy. A typical set of iMRI images used for targeting is shown on the panel monitor behind the surgeon.

A fusion, or overlay, of these images is used to determine the most dopamine-depleted regions of the putamen that would make the most ideal cell transplantation targets. This preoperative surgical planning should be useful to determine the number of cells to be used and the number of brain penetrations required.

Confirmation that dopaminergic precursor cells are healthy and available for transplantation. This confirmation includes cellular and molecular analysis, some of which is performed the day before surgery. The dissociated cell suspension is also examined by study personnel on the day of surgery before the patient is placed under general anesthesia.

Induction of anesthesia and positioning of the patient on the MRI gantry. After general anesthesia is induced, the patient is positioned supine on the MRI gantry. The patient's head is mounted in a MR-compatible (eg, carbon-fiber) headholder, which is mounted on the gantry. After MR surface coils are positioned around the head, the gantry is moved into the magnet so that the head is at the MRI field isocenter.

Preliminary target determination. A volumetric, gadolinium-enhanced MRI is obtained, and initial targets are selected. Fusion of the MRI images to the PD-PET scan may be useful to correlate the preoperative plan (from step 1 above) to this first iMRI scan. These preliminary targets are only used for trajectory planning (see article by Starr and colleagues elsewhere in this issue for details).

Determination of burr hole location. iMRI fluoroscopy is then used to determine the trajectory entry point. This point is marked on the scalp.

Preparation of sterile field, creation of burr hole, and placement of the trajectory guide device. For the purposes of this outline, we envision the use of a device similar to the Nexframe DBA (deep brain access) (Medtronic, Minneapolis, Minnesota) trajectory guide as described elsewhere in this issue. To increase access to the patient's head, the gantry is slid through the center of the magnet, allowing the surgeon to work outside of the confines of the magnet. At the marked location (from step 5 above), the scalp is opened, a burr hole created, dura and pia opened, and the DBA device is mounted.

Reimaging after burr hole and mounting of the DBA device. The patient is returned to the magnet isocenter, and no further table movements are made until after cells are delivered into the brain. To compensate for brain shift that occurs after introduction of air and loss of cerebral spinal fluid through the burr hole, a new iMRI scan is obtained. A new, precise trajectory is determined from this second iMRI scan, and, using the MR fluoroscopy sequence, the surgeon then lines up the targeting device with the anatomic target.

Placement of cell delivery guide cannula. The surgeon then introduces the MR-compatible cannula for cell delivery. This procedure is monitored with MR fluoroscopy.

Confirmation of cannula location at the intended target. After the cannula has been lowered to the target, a limited MRI sequence is obtained to confirm that the cannula is indeed at the intended anatomic location.

Transplantation of cells. Cells are then delivered through the cannula. The actual design of the cannula (eg, side ports versus end port) and method of injection can be adapted to this overall procedure as long as MR-compatible tools and devices are used.

Removal of cannula, repositioning to new trajectory, and delivery of cells to other intended targets (repeat of steps 7–11).

At the end of procedure, another MRI is obtained to document cell transplant locations (if cells are labeled with an MR contrast agent) and assess for potential surgical complications (eg, hemorrhage).

## SUMMARY

In the near future, we will likely see clinical trials testing the use of hESC-derived dopaminergic neurons for the treatment of PD. As exciting as this prospect is, we do recognize that there are many issues that must be considered if we are to obtain satisfactory, long-term treatment of PD. It has now become almost standard to transplant neurons into the dopamine-depleted putamen for PD; however, the initial loss of neurons occurs in the substantia nigra pars compacta (SNc). Perhaps the SNc is a better target for dopaminergic neuron transplantation. After all, one common goal of the cell biologist has been to produce a population of so-called "A9 neurons" whose cell bodies actually belong in the SNc and not the putamen. It is possible that these A9 neurons would survive better in the native environment of the SNc. The challenge then is to induce such neurons grafted to the SNc to project axons over long distances to the normal anatomic targets. We hope that the biologic understanding necessary to accomplish such "rewiring" of damaged circuits progresses rapidly to the point that recapitulating these processes in the adult brain will be possible. Axonal projections from the SNc to physiologically relevant areas may reduce the incidence of GIDs (by avoiding excessive, aberrant intrastriatal dopaminergic innervation produced by putaminal grafts) and allow other reinnervations (eg, to the pedunculopontine nucleus,

which may aid in the recovery of posture and balance in addition to the motor benefits). Furthermore, it is even possible that other nonmotor symptoms of PD (eg, decreased cognition) may be alleviated by transplants to the SNc or nonmotor regions of the putamen. iMRI as a surgical technology will be helpful in achieving the accurate placement of cells to the relatively small and deep structures of the brain, including the SNc. We believe that iMRI cell transplantation techniques can be easily modified to target a multitude of different brain regions for various neurologic disorders, including stroke, Alzheimer disease, and multiple sclerosis.

## REFERENCES

1. Jellinger K. New developments in the pathology of Parkinson's disease. Adv Neurol 1990;53:1–16.

2. Kish SJ, Shannak K, Hornykiewicz O. Uneven pattern of dopamine loss in the striatum of patients with idiopathic Parkinson's disease. Pathophysiologic and clinical implications. N Engl J Med 1988; 318:876–80.

3. Brooks DJ, Salmon EP, Mathias CJ, et al. The relationship between locomotor disability, autonomic dysfunction, and the integrity of the striatal dopaminergic system in patients with multiple system atrophy, pure autonomic failure, and Parkinson's disease, studied with PET. Brain 1990;113(Pt 5): 1539–52.

4. Cotzias GC, Van Woert MH, Schiffer LM. Aromatic amino acids and modification of parkinsonism. N Engl J Med 1967;276:374–9.

5. Marsden CD, Parkes JD. "On-off" effects in patients with Parkinson's disease on chronic levodopa therapy. Lancet 1976;1:292–6.

6. Marsden CD, Parkes JD. Success and problems of long-term levodopa therapy in Parkinson's disease. Lancet 1977;1:345–9.

7. Lindvall O, Brundin P, Widner H, et al. Grafts of fetal dopamine neurons survive and improve motor function in Parkinson's disease. Science 1990;247:574–7.

8. Piccini P, Lindvall O, Bjorklund A, et al. Delayed recovery of movement-related cortical function in Parkinson's disease after striatal dopaminergic grafts. Ann Neurol 2000;48:689–95.

9. Piccini P, Brooks DJ, Bjorklund A, et al. Dopamine release from nigral transplants visualized in vivo in a Parkinson's patient. Nat Neurosci 1999;2:1137–40.

10. Winkler C, Kirik D, Bjorklund A. Cell transplantation in Parkinson's disease: how can we make it work? Trends Neurosci 2005;28:86–92.

11. Freed CR, Greene PE, Breeze RE, et al. Transplantation of embryonic dopamine neurons for severe Parkinson's disease. N Engl J Med 2001;344:710–9.

12. Olanow CW, Goetz CG, Kordower JH, et al. A double-blind controlled trial of bilateral fetal nigral transplantation in Parkinson's disease. Ann Neurol 2003;54:403–14.

13. Choong C, Rao MS. Human embryonic stem cells. Neurosurg Clin N Am 2007;18:1–14, vii.

14. Deierborg T, Soulet D, Roybon L, et al. Emerging restorative treatments for Parkinson's disease. Prog Neurobiol 2008;85:407–32.

15. Kim JH, Auerbach JM, Rodriguez-Gomez JA, et al. Dopamine neurons derived from embryonic stem cells function in an animal model of Parkinson's disease. Nature 2002;418:50–6.

16. Brederlau A, Correia AS, Anisimov SV, et al. Transplantation of human embryonic stem cell-derived cells to a rat model of Parkinson's disease: effect of in vitro differentiation on graft survival and teratoma formation. Stem Cells 2006;24:1433–40.

17. Buytaert-Hoefen KA, Alvarez E, Freed CR. Generation of tyrosine hydroxylase positive neurons from human embryonic stem cells after coculture with cellular substrates and exposure to GDNF. Stem Cells 2004;22:669–74.

18. Chiba S, Lee YM, Zhou W, et al. Noggin enhances dopamine neuron production from human embryonic stem cells and improves behavioral outcome after transplantation into Parkinsonian rats. Stem Cells 2008;26:2810–20.

19. Cho MS, Lee YE, Kim JY, et al. Highly efficient and large-scale generation of functional dopamine neurons from human embryonic stem cells. Proc Natl Acad Sci U S A 2008;105:3392–7.

20. Park CH, Minn YK, Lee JY, et al. In vitro and in vivo analyses of human embryonic stem cell-derived dopamine neurons. J Neurochem 2005;92:1265–76.

21. Park S, Lee KS, Lee YJ, et al. Generation of dopaminergic neurons in vitro from human embryonic stem cells treated with neurotrophic factors. Neurosci Lett 2004;359:99–103.

22. Perrier AL, Tabar V, Barberi T, et al. Derivation of midbrain dopamine neurons from human embryonic stem cells. Proc Natl Acad Sci U S A 2004;101:12543–8.

23. Roy NS, Cleren C, Singh SK, et al. Functional engraftment of human ES cell-derived dopaminergic neurons enriched by coculture with telomerase-immortalized midbrain astrocytes. Nat Med 2006;12:1259–68.

24. Schulz TC, Noggle SA, Palmarini GM, et al. Differentiation of human embryonic stem cells to dopaminergic neurons in serum-free suspension culture. Stem Cells 2004;22:1218–38.

25. Sonntag KC, Pruszak J, Yoshizaki T, et al. Enhanced yield of neuroepithelial precursors and midbrain-like dopaminergic neurons from human embryonic stem cells using the bone morphogenic protein antagonist noggin. Stem Cells 2007;25:411–8.

26. Ueno M, Matsumura M, Watanabe K, et al. Neural conversion of ES cells by an inductive activity on human amniotic membrane matrix. Proc Natl Acad Sci U S A 2006;103:9554–9.

27. Yan Y, Yang D, Zarnowska ED, et al. Directed differentiation of dopaminergic neuronal subtypes from human embryonic stem cells. Stem Cells 2005;23:781–90.

28. Zeng X, Cai J, Chen J, et al. Dopaminergic differentiation of human embryonic stem cells. Stem Cells 2004;22:925–40.

29. Tabar V, Tomishima M, Panagiotakos G, et al. Therapeutic cloning in individual parkinsonian mice. Nat Med 2008;14:379–81.

30. Wernig M, Zhao JP, Pruszak J, et al. Neurons derived from reprogrammed fibroblasts functionally integrate into the fetal brain and improve symptoms of rats with Parkinson's disease. Proc Natl Acad Sci U S A 2008;105:5856–61.

31. Kordower JH, Chu Y, Hauser RA, et al. Lewy body-like pathology in long-term embryonic nigral transplants in Parkinson's disease. Nat Med 2008;14:504–6.

32. Li JY, Englund E, Holton JL, et al. Lewy bodies in grafted neurons in subjects with Parkinson's disease suggest host-to-graft disease propagation. Nat Med 2008;14:501–3.

33. Mendez I, Vinuela A, Astradsson A, et al. Dopamine neurons implanted into people with Parkinson's disease survive without pathology for 14 years. Nat Med 2008;14:507–9.

34. Subramanian T, Deogaonkar M, Brummer M, et al. MRI guidance improves accuracy of stereotaxic targeting for cell transplantation in parkinsonian monkeys. Exp Neurol 2005;193:172–80.

35. Tsao K, Wilkinson S, Overman J, et al. Comparison of actual pallidotomy lesion location with expected stereotactic location. Stereotact Funct Neurosurg 1998;71:1–19.

36. Bourgeois G, Magnin M, Morel A, et al. Accuracy of MRI-guided stereotactic thalamic functional neurosurgery. Neuroradiology 1999;41:636–45.

37. Bejjani BP, Dormont D, Pidoux B, et al. Bilateral subthalamic stimulation for Parkinson's disease by using three-dimensional stereotactic magnetic resonance imaging and electrophysiological guidance. J Neurosurg 2000;92:615–25.

38. Cuny E, Guehl D, Burbaud P, et al. Lack of agreement between direct magnetic resonance imaging and statistical determination of a subthalamic target: the role of electrophysiological guidance. J Neurosurg 2002;97:591–7.

39. Starr PA, Christine CW, Theodosopoulos PV, et al. Implantation of deep brain stimulators into the subthalamic nucleus: technical approach and magnetic resonance imaging-verified lead locations. J Neurosurg 2002;97:370–87.

40. Ma Y, Feigin A, Dhawan V, et al. Dyskinesia after fetal cell transplantation for parkinsonism: a PET study. Ann Neurol 2002;52:628–34.

41. Breeze RE, Wells TH Jr, Freed CR. Implantation of fetal tissue for the management of Parkinson's disease: a technical note. Neurosurgery 1995;36: 1044–7 [discussion: 1047–8].

42. Mendez I, Hong M, Smith S, et al. Neural transplantation cannula and microinjector system: experimental and clinical experience. Technical note. J Neurosurg 2000;92:493–9.

43. Slotkin JR, Cahill KS, Tharin SA, et al. Cellular magnetic resonance imaging: nanometer and micrometer size particles for noninvasive cell localization. Neurotherapeutics 2007;4:428–33.

44. Shapiro EM, Koretsky AP. Convertible manganese contrast for molecular and cellular MRI. Magn Reson Med 2008;60:265–9.

# Erratum

In the October 2008 issue of *Neurosurgery Clinics of North America*, the affiliations listed for the authors of *Magnetic Resonance Imaging of Peripheral Nerves* were incorrect.

Dr. Amrami and Dr. Felmlee were incorrectly identified as affiliated with the Division of Magnetic Resonance Imaging. They are both affiliated with the Department of Radiology, Mayo Clinic, 200 1st Street SW, Rochester, MN 55905, USA.

Dr. Spinner was incorrectly identified as affiliated with the Department of Radiology. He is affiliated solely with the Department of Neurologic Surgery, Mayo Clinic, 200 1st Street SW, Rochester, MN 55905, USA.

Neurosurg Clin N Am 20 (2009) 233
doi:10.1016/j.nec.2008.12.001
1042-3680/08/$ – see front matter © 2009 Elsevier Inc. All rights reserved.

Neurosurg Clin N Am 21 (2010) 221
doi:10.1016/j.nec.2009.12.001
1042-3680/10/$ – see front matter © 2009 Elsevier Inc. All rights reserved.

# Index

*Note:* Page numbers of article titles are in **boldface** type.

Neurosurg Clin N Am 20 (2009) 235–237
doi:10.1016/S1042-3680(09)00029-1

# Moving?

## Make sure your subscription moves with you!

To notify us of your new address, find your **Clinics Account Number** (located on your mailing label above your name), and contact customer service at:

**E-mail: elspcs@elsevier.com**

**800-654-2452 (subscribers in the U.S. & Canada)**
**314-453-7041 (subscribers outside of the U.S. & Canada)**

**Fax number: 314-523-5170**

**Elsevier Periodicals Customer Service**
11830 Westline Industrial Drive
St. Louis, MO 63146

*To ensure uninterrupted delivery of your subscription, please notify us at least 4 weeks in advance of move.

ELSEVIER

Printed and bound by CPI Group (UK) Ltd, Croydon, CR0 4YY

03/10/2024

01040361-0002